Praise for *Superior Vocal Health*

"Not only does David have an extraordinary voice and a remarkable life story, he cares about people and is dedicated to the natural approach to living, singing and healing. This is the kind of simple, thorough handbook, or bible if you will that all of us singers have been waiting for. I'll be packing this in my tour bag from now on."

—TONY HARNELL
(critically acclaimed, award winning rock vocalist)
www.tonyharnell.com

I have never before seen such a concise yet comprehensive presentation of natural remedies for vocal health, along with such specific directions for using them! Katz' book is one I will recommend to all my vocal students and recording/ performing artists. I fully expect my singers and public speakers to include a copy in their briefcases and road luggage, along with a protective stash of some of the remedies suggested. I won't leave home without it, myself!

—JUDY RODMAN, professional vocal coach, recording producer, public speaker, singer, performer

David Katz's new book, Superior Vocal Health, is a landmark resource for singers all over the world. His thorough knowledge and application of herbal remedies that will promote vocal vibrancy is unmatched. His recovery from serious illness and near vocal collapse is an inspiration of hope for anyone who is struggling with health issues that affect their voice. This book should be every serious singer's constant companion.

—KATHRYNE PIRTLE, Clarinetist, Orion Ensemble, Author, *Performance Without Pain* (New Trends, 2006), *Acid Reflux: Achieving Lasting Healing with Traditional Foods* (E-book, 2009)

I have used David's products for 2 years now, daily, for prevention and symtom relief. My patients have used the products successfully. Now with this fantastic book, I have a better way to educate my students and patients about their Vocal Health. It is a concise guide and p!

D1518207

teachers, singers, and parents today. More importantly this seeds the future of Vocal Health on this planet.

—DR. BARRY J. GOODMAN, Chiropractor, Reiki Master, Yogic
Neuromuscular Therapy
http://www.aquarianyahh.org

Courtroom lawyers are no where without a healthy and powerful vocal instrument. This book is an amazing resource and must have item for lawyers everywhere,. Pass it on!

—KAREN SMOLAR,
Trial Chief, The Bronx Defenders, New York

SUPERIOR VOCAL

HEALTH

HERBS FOR THE VOICE AND THROAT

*A Guide to Herbs,
Supplements, and Diet for
the Voice Professional*

David Aaron Katz

Vendera
Publishing

Cover and Interior Design: Daniel Middleton
www.scribefreelance.com

ISBN: 978-1-936307-27-2

Printed in the United States of America

This book is dedicated to every single Voice Professional on this planet. All of those people who strive to use their voice and gifts to the best of their ability, enriching, inspiring and uplifting all who hear them.

I would also like to thank those people who helped make this book a reality: My wife Julia, and daughters Rayna and Hanna. Your endless care and inquiry: "Is your book done yet?" helped push me to achieve my dream.

Fred Mollin and Jaime Babbitt for your endless support and help.

Jaime Vendera for your guidance and continual "friendly pressure" to get the job done.

Jimmy Webb, Judy Rodman, Tony Harnell, Guruganesha Singh and all the other incredible artists who use and endorse Superior Vocal Health formulas to take care of their voices.

Kathryne Pirtle and Judy Rodman for your professional guidance and friendship.

Stuart Kahan, for your endless guidance, advice, and mentoring without ever asking for anything in return. Bob Binder for his wonderful recipes, guidance and never ending support.

Brian Reardon for his inspiration and friendship encouraging the continued growth of Superior Vocal Health.

My mother Judith, thank you.

*My brother Evan, for inspiring me with his
courage and will to live.
And his daughter, my niece, Sarah,
for loving me so sweetly.*

CONTENTS

INTRODUCTION 8

CHAPTER ONE: My Personal Story 11

CHAPTER TWO: The Voice Professional's Herbal Medicine Chest 16

   Specific Herbs and Their Uses 17

CHAPTER THREE: Specific Herbal Formulas 60

   Allergy and Sinus Congestion Formulas 60
   Cold and Flu Formulas 61
   Energy and Endurance Formulas 62
   Hoarseness, Laryngitis and Overused, Tired Voice Formulas 63
   Chest and Lung Formulas 64
   Immune Boosting Formulas 64
   Nerve, Anxiety and Sleep Formulas 65

CHAPTER FOUR: Sinus Health 68

   General Usage for the Neti Pot 68

CHAPTER FIVE: Prescription Medication, Drugs and Their Effects on the Throat and Voice 70

CHAPTER SIX: Natural Food Supplements 75

   Allergies 75
   Brain Function, Memory and Alertness 76
   Bronchial and Respiratory 77
   Energy and Fatigue 78
   Immune System Boosting 79
   Nerves and the Nervous System 80

CHAPTER SEVEN: On-the-Run Foods for the Voice Professional 82

CHAPTER EIGHT: Proper Acid/Alkaline Balance 90

CHAPTER NINE: What Do I Do When? 93

INTRODUCTION

Hello, my name is David Aaron Katz. I'm a voice professional. This means my entire life revolves around and depends upon the health of my voice. If I have a sore throat, sinus congestion, sinusitis, asthma, phlegm, a tired or overused voice, or the flu and cannot perform, my career and financial livelihood are at stake.

When your voice is the way in which you earn income, you must protect your instrument. Still, this book is invaluable for all because most likely, in some form or another, the majority of us use our voices throughout our day job. Whether you are a singer, actor, broadcaster, clergy, teacher, professional speaker, public speaker, politician, salesperson, church soloist, singer in a band, nightclub singer or tour guide, vocal health should be the most important concern in your life.

We are not like the athlete, financial planner, writer, administrator, mechanic, or computer programmer who can do their job when sick. Singers and speakers are in dire consequences when our throat and voice becomes weak and/or damaged. When our voice sounds weak, unfortunately WE are perceived as weak, or less powerful. In fact, we are almost always judged by our last performance, presentation, sermon, or tour no matter what our track record may show. We must be in absolute top vocal form every single day for every performance, no matter what our life situation happens to be.

I believe we can always be in superior vocal health no matter what the situation. At this point you might be thinking to yourself, "Are you telling me that you never get sick, David?" The answer is, "Rarely." Since I began using the herbs, supplements and food suggestions in this book, I do not have vocal health issues anymore in my life. The truth of the matter is that the only time I did have a sore throat, cold, chest affliction, or phlegm is when I didn't follow the guidelines and suggestions in this book.

We as voice professionals cannot afford to have any vocal or throat issues. Stop right here and re-read the previous sentence three times out loud. Your voice depends on it. Therefore, we must find a way to stay on top vocally every day of our life. I believe this is possible for everyone, because I personally experience this level of superior vocal health myself.

There are no coincidences in life. You are reading this book for a reason. You are a voice professional who wants to be at your very best. Lucky for you, you now have in your hands one of the most important tools you will ever have in your vocal tool box. *Superior Vocal Health* is the voice professional's guide to maintaining superior vocal health naturally, without chemicals or drugs. It is a simple, easy to use guidebook that will teach you how to naturally maintain your voice (throat) and entire body at optimal levels. This will not only improve your voice, but your overall health will also benefit from these choices. You will know exactly what to do for any situation that comes up. Whether you are on the road, at home or touring the world, this book will be your saving grace. Keep it with you wherever you go.

Of course, some vocal problems such as nodules, cancer, laryngeal thrush, acid reflux or GERD, and other physical issues may be present that will make your road to superior vocal health more challenging. I'm not a doctor, and I'm not in any way claiming to diagnose or treat vocal problems which may be due to inadequate training, lack of proper technique, or abuse of the vocal cords and entire body.

Poor technique is another issue altogether and one that I am not addressing in this book. My assumption is that you, as a voice professional, take your craft very seriously and have worked on vocal technique. You understand that your entire life depends on the absolute top quality care of your throat and voice at all times.

My goal is to provide you with the tools that will allow you to come to understand and accept that optimal vocal health and voice production are entirely possible as well as the most important things in your entire life. My wish is that you experience for yourself the gift I have received in my life as an Opera singer, Cantor, teacher, coach, and lecturer, which is the gift of Superior Vocal Health.

So, without further ado let us begin our journey toward Superior Vocal Health!

Disclaimer: The following sections and statement have not been evaluated by the FDA and are not intended to prescribe, treat, prevent or diagnose any disease or illness. Consult your physician before taking any of the listed food products, vitamins, minerals, or herbs.

CHAPTER ONE
MY PERSONAL STORY

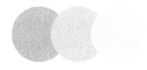

I have been singing professionally for the last 25 years. I've always been obsessed with how the voice works and how to improve my voice. Early in my career I was not affected by my unhealthy lifestyle choices. I was in decent health, exercised regularly, and kept my voice well-oiled with weekly study.

Then all of a sudden something happened...Life! I got married, had children, and was working full time as a Cantor and singer. I was teaching, training choirs, and studying regularly twice a week with my vocal and repertoire coaches in Manhattan, New York. I was commuting on a train full of people who were coughing, sneezing and such. I was also working with children on a regular basis. To say the least, I was using my voice constantly, pushing it to the most extreme levels to continually perform and produce under challenging circumstances. At the same time, I was doing auditions for major opera companies and whatever other jobs I could land. Many times I would get the job and then find myself commuting an additional two days a week for rehearsals. Of course we can't forget the family responsibilities either! Sound familiar?

All of this would not have been so bad had I not been living the abusive, debilitating diet of the average American, which consisted of dangerously high caffeine consumption, addiction to white sugar, white flour, white salt and empty carbohydrates combined with large amounts of dairy and processed meats. This diet was slowly killing me and destroying my voice.

Throughout this experience, I was always super careful about doing vocal exercises every day and trying my best to not abuse my voice. This was out of fear, because I never forgot what one of my first managers in New York said to me as a young singer:

"David, your voice must always be in top form, because I may call you at any time of the day or night with an audition or performance. I will not accept you telling me you are tired or

can't make it because you aren't vocally in shape. If you want to
play in the big leagues, you need to always be ready to sing."

Luckily, I had outstanding training and had worked hard. I was able to keep my voice in decent shape and hide most of the ragged feeling I was experiencing in my throat. Because the bottom line is that for every great singer who gets a job, there are thousands more just as good standing right outside the door. So I never wanted to let on to any stage director, conductor, or agent that my voice was tired, my cords were slightly roughed up, or that I "needed a break." This, I had decided, was professional suicide, and I was not willing to risk losing the work or develop a reputation as a singer who was inconsistent, unreliable, or could not perform when needed.

When I did happen to get sick, which was every four months or so on a regular basis, I just slammed into my body whatever I could get my hands on. I have probably taken every antibiotic on the planet! I also was a full time user of all the over-the-counter decongestants and cold medicines on the market, as well as a connoisseur of OTC sleep aids. In addition, due to genetics and hereditary issues, I was on three major pharmaceutical drugs for more than 15 years for everything from depression and anxiety to attention deficit disorder! (Hmm, I wonder if my diet had anything to do with all of this!!!)

Then in the middle of what I thought was a normal singer's lifestyle, I became seriously ill. Out of nowhere (I like to say it this way because today it makes me laugh as if it happened by chance!) I felt like I got hit by the worst flu I had ever experienced. Within 20 minutes, I was lying in bed shaking uncontrollably, convulsing, and freezing with chills. My body felt as if someone had hammered nails into every joint. I had the worst digestive cramping I had ever experienced in my life. I could not lie still in one position for more than 15 seconds due to the intense pain in my gut and throughout my body. Naturally, the first thing I did was have my wife drive me to the 24- hour clinic to get a fresh batch of antibiotics. However, this time it was much worse and I was rushed to the emergency room.

As I waited for a room, the pain became so intense and I was screaming out so much, the doctors literally shot me up with morphine just so I could sit still and my body could rest. The next few days were a blur. I had endless needles in me pumping liquid nutrients and antibiotics into my body. I couldn't eat or drink anything. My colon was so damaged that when I tried eating, I vomited, my stomach cramped up or I had intense diarrhea. I remember having to prepare myself for a colonoscopy. I couldn't even hold myself up because I was so weak. I crawled into the bathroom in the hospital room, laid down on the cold floor and gave myself an enema. The pain was unbelievable.

After the results of the colonoscopy, the doctors told me that I had some difficult digestive "issues" and a few days after the next round antibiotics kicked in I would be fine. No one told me what was wrong or what had happened, except that my colon had taken a beating; possibly Crohns or some other digestive disease, but nothing concrete. They gave me more medication and sent me home two days later. I won't lie, I did feel slightly better. I could hold down a small amount of food, but not much because I still had massive digestive cramps and diarrhea almost every time I ate or drank anything.

Over the next few weeks, I went back to work and slowly resumed the same diet I had been eating before. After all, no doctor even addressed what I had been putting into my body, so why do anything different? As I resumed my typical diet, albeit in small portions, the symptoms worsened again. I ended up losing almost 20 pounds in the next few weeks. I looked gaunt and my ribs and collarbone were starting to show. The scariest part of it all through the entire experience was that my voice began to take a serious beating. It was, at the most, half of what it used to be. I could not even support my sound because I had become so weak. The muscles around my diaphragm felt so abused from endless vomiting and cramping that I could barely access them for singing.

I followed up with my doctor to tell him what I was experiencing on a daily basis. He said, "If you have diarrhea one more time, you need to get in here immediately because we are going to have to cut out the portion of your colon that is experiencing problems, which means you will probably have to wear a bag for the rest of your life."

I was devastated mentally, physically, and spiritually. As I lay in bed that night staring up at the ceiling I said to myself, "David, you feel like dying. Your colon is destroyed and you are in the beginning of a very promising career. What the hell is going on?"

Thus began the beginning of what I now call my "new life." The very next day, a vocal coach who was a dear friend called to see how I was doing. I told her the news and she asked me one question that changed my life. "Are you ready to take control and responsibility of your voice, career, and ultimately your life?" Without hesitation I said yes and asked her what should be done. She gave me the name of one of the best Natural Doctors and Chinese Doctors in New York. I booked an appointment and soon learned that my colon had small tears due to an abuse of antibiotics and pharmaceuticals. All the content that normally filters out of the body through feces was slowly seeping into my bloodstream and literally poisoning me to death.

Over the course of the following month, I saw these doctors two to three times per week. We began to slowly and systematically cleanse my body of the toxins that had nearly destroyed my colon. By month two I could eat regularly, was gaining weight again, and my strength was slowly coming back to me.

Thus began my life as a man obsessed with taking care of my vocal health, personal health, and family's health, all naturally without chemicals or drugs. Over the next year, I held fast to a strict diet that my new doctors and nutritionists gave me. At the end of that first year, something happened once again that changed my life. My voice had come back full force and actually sounded as though it had doubled in size. It was clearer and more powerful than I had ever experienced, and there was a vibrancy and ring that had never been there before. It was then that I realized the total connection between my body's health and the health of my voice: What you put into your body directly affects the health of your voice, and in my case ultimately my career.

A few years later, I was so inspired that I decided to become a nutritional consultant and herbalist. Although I had been using various herbs throughout my career, this experience had inspired me to begin using more herbs, supplements, and follow a strict diet to maintain superior vocal health.

This was the beginning of my research and personal experience with how to heal, strengthen, and maintain my voice naturally. I researched all the herbs that directly helped heal the issues that voice professionals deal with on a regular basis, including clogged sinuses, mucus buildup in the throat, chest, and vocal cords, respiratory issues, energy, mental clarity, relaxation, and sleep. The result of this research and experience is what you are now holding in your hands.

So, if you are ready to accept responsibility for your own voice and career, turn to the next chapter and give yourself the gift of *Superior Vocal Health*.

CHAPTER TWO
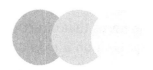
THE VOICE PROFESSIONAL'S HERBAL MEDICINE CHEST

In this book, I've put together what I feel to be the singer's herbal medicine chest. Herbs come in many forms, once taken out of their raw form as plants. For ease of use and need, I will not go into all the forms herbs can be used. My suggestions below are primarily for use as liquid extracts, capsules, or teas. The reason for this is obvious: Very few voice professionals are herbalists, and most of us do not have the time or energy to "prepare" formulas. Herbal extracts, capsules, and teas provide some of the fastest and most powerful ways to get the results we need.

An herbal extract is a liquid solvent in which the main ingredient of an herb powder becomes soluble. Herb powder is put through a special cold extraction process. This allows the herb to percolate cold with suitable solvents for each herb. Water, grape brandy, alcohol, and apple cider vinegar are the most commonly used solvents, either alone or in combination. For singers, it is best to stay away from alcohol-based herbs because alcohol can dry out the vocal cords.

Extracts are the most preferred choice for ingesting herbs because they are easier to take than pills or capsules. They can be mixed with water (or any other preferred liquid) or placed directly on or under the tongue. They absorb into your system faster and more efficiently for some people who may have digestion issues or poor absorption. Extracts are also preferred by children as they may have difficulty swallowing pills or capsules.

The following list of herbs is by no means all inclusive, but extremely comprehensive in its content regarding accessible herbs that can help promote healing, strengthen the voice, and assist with many voice related issues that voice professionals deal with on a regular basis.

Note: All of the listed herbs can be used in capsule form, extract, or tea unless noted otherwise. Also note that throughout this book, various herbs, supplements, and foods may be repeated due to their many uses; this is because many of the herbs mentioned can help treat the same ailment or illness. However, not everyone reacts the same way to each herb or combination, As you try different herbal combinations, pay close attention to how your body reacts to each so you will know which herbs benefit you the most.

SPECIFIC HERBS AND THEIR USES

Herbs and herbal combinations work in conjunction with your body to help stimulate and support your body's natural healing system. I've listed specific herbs that are useful in healing, maintaining, strengthening, treating, and supporting the throat, vocal cords, throat muscles, nasal cavity and passages, chest cavity, brain, nervous system, and overall body, with the ultimate goal being the attainment of superior vocal health.

When using herbs to heal and strengthen the voice and body, it is very important to understand that every "body" is different, unique, and will react differently to certain herbs and dosage levels. Herbs are not chemicals. They must be taken consistently and for extended periods of time to work effectively and do the job. Use them wisely and with proper instruction, and allow the time needed to heal. Thoroughly read each of the following herbal descriptions before choosing where to start on your path to superior vocal health.

Alfalfa

Alfalfa is an energy booster used by many athletes for endurance. Native Americans were known to feed their horses alfalfa to make them run faster, and to their cows so they might produce more milk. Due to the roots extending more than 20 feet into the ground, alfalfa is full of trace minerals and nutrients which help alkalize and detoxify the entire body. Alfalfa also contains many highly needed digestive enzymes. It is very useful in treating fevers and is a good source of chlorophyll. To take advantage of and receive the most benefit from all of its nutrients, vitamins and minerals, eat alfalfa in its sprouted state. If you are unable to get raw sprouts, raw powder form is also effective and can easily be mixed with juice or water for a tasty drink.

It is truly a super food containing vitamins A, B1, B6, B12, C, E, and K1, as well as essential amino acids.

Aloe
Aloe is most commonly used as a topical agent for relieving burns and sores. When taken internally, it can be used to soothe stomach irritation. It is excellent for reducing and eliminating mucus and debris from the stomach, liver, kidneys, spleen and bladder. It is one of the best body cleansers known and has been shown to be an excellent immune booster. Taken in small doses of 1/4 teaspoon daily, it will help keep the digestive system healthy and clean, reducing acid reflux and other digestive difficulties. Taking aloe can also help with a cough, and it can be used as a gargle for a sore throat due to its ability to help injured tissues in the body.

> **Note:** Most herbalists do not recommend taking Aloe internally when pregnant, as it may induce abortion and stimulate menstruation.

Alum Root
Alum Root is highly effective in relieving sore throats, especially when made into a tea or used in extract form as a gargle. Due to its powerful astringent properties, it is also used as a mouthwash for bleeding gums and mouth sores. For use of swollen or inflamed gums, brew a strong tea of Alum and rinse the mouth up to three times per day. Do not swallow. Spit out the mixture after rinsing. To make a brew of Alum tea, add two tablespoons of fresh alum powder to one pint of boiling water in a small to medium sized cooking pot. Allow the herb to boil for three minutes. Take off heat and steep with the pot covered for 20 minutes. Strain and let sit to cool. Drink hot or warm. This may be used for a sore throat as well.

> **Note:** Alum Root can cause gastrointestinal irritation if taken in large amounts. Most herbalists do not recommend exceeding more than one cup per day and to not use for more than three days in a row.

Angelica

In the middle ages, Angelica was considered to have magical powers to protect the user against evil of all kinds. In Chinese medicine, Angelica has been used for thousands of years to treat female issues. Angelica is a fine remedy for stomach issues, heartburn and cramps. It is also excellent for relief of bronchitis, coughs, sore throat, colds and other respiratory conditions because of its expectorant qualities. It has been noted to contain anti-inflammatory properties useful for reducing swelling as well as helping to lower fevers. Taken as a hot tea, it can break up mucus in the throat and lungs quickly. Put two tablespoons in one pint of boiling water. Boil for three to five minutes. Take off heat, let sit covered for 15 minutes, strain and drink. Drink three to four cups throughout the day for up to three days when fighting respiratory symptoms.

Note: Most herbalists do not recommend taking Angelica by anyone who is pregnant as it can cause uterine contractions.

Anise

Anise is considered a multi-purpose tea because of its purported ability to help deal with oily skin and improve memory. Anise also aids digestion, clears mucus from the air passages, and combats respiratory infections including sinusitis. It is an excellent agent to help with gas, nausea, and acid reflux because it balances out the stomach acids thus reducing the conditions that accompany acid reflux. Chewing the raw seeds after a meal can help alleviate indigestion as well as sweeten the breath. It is also used in commercial cough medicines because its flavor resembles licorice. For a strong and powerful tea add three tablespoons of seed to five cups of boiling water. Take off heat and let sit covered for 10 minutes. Strain and drink. Drink up to four cups a day for one week for stubborn coughs.

Note: Most herbalists do not recommend taking Anise while pregnant as it has the ability to induce abortion.

Ashwagandha

Ashwagandha is an herb that is highly revered in Ayurvedic, Siddah and Unami medicine. Ashwagandha is an outstanding herb for combating stress because it is an adaptogen that helps to adjust the body's response to stress. Ashwagandha rejuvenates and energizes the entire nervous system as well as strengthens the immune system. It has anti-inflammatory properties which may help to reduce swelling in the throat. It is also used to increase physical endurance, strength, and energy. In addition, it has been shown to improve sexual function. One to two capsules daily (if you are undergoing more stress than normal) is effective in combating stress and giving your body the support it needs. Ashwagandha may also be taken effectively as a liquid extract when mixed with Ginger or green tea. One dropper per cup of tea is excellent for sustained energy in the morning to start your day, or before a concert or presentation.

Note: Due to its high iron content and possibilities of inducing abortion, most herbalists do not recommend taking Ashwagandha during pregnancy with alcohol or anti-anxiety drugs.

Astragalus

Astragalus is a highly regarded herb in Chinese medicine used for all sorts of ailments that cause a person to feel lackluster or exhausted. It is an excellent herb when used for an energy boost, increasing total body vitality and resistance to disease by bolstering the immune system. It is used by athletes for overall body energy and maintaining energy reserves. When combined with ginseng, it works as a complete body energizer both inside and out. This herb can easily replace caffeine when used regularly, with none of the side effects that accompany caffeine consumption. Astragalus increases stamina and is good for colds, flu, and upper respiratory infections. Astragalus can be taken in capsule form or liquid extract. A full dropper in ginseng tea provides excellent support and energy when you know you have a long rehearsal or traveling to a performance. Two capsules in the morning are very effective for providing energy throughout the day.

Note: Most herbalists do not recommend taking Astragalus when fever is present, as it may make the fever last longer and possibly grow stronger.

Barley Grass

Barley Grass is an excellent source for almost all the vitamins and minerals needed to maintain a healthy and vibrant body. Roman Gladiators were known to eat the grass for strength and stamina. Barley Grass has also been shown to help those with gluten allergies because of its high content of chlorophyll. For those who do not wish to consume dairy products to avoid mucus buildup in the throat and body but still want their calcium, an eight-ounce cup of raw Barley Grass juice contains 10 times the calcium found in milk. Barley Grass has been used for years in soothing sore throats due to its demulcent properties. For an excellent barley tea, heat (do not boil) 1/2 cup of barley grass in three cups of water for 10 minutes. Strain and drink either warm or cold.

Bayberry

Bayberry tea is an excellent gargle when used for any kind of sore throat. It will completely cleanse the throat of all unwanted and debilitating debris. When consumed as a warm tea, it will promote perspiration improving the entire circulation. Bayberry can be used as a snuff for nasal congestion and sinus problems. It improves circulation and has laxative properties. For an outstanding cold formula that contains bayberry, see the formula section under "colds." To use as a tea, add one tablespoon of fresh bayberry herb to three cups of water and boil for 10 minutes. Take off heat an let sit covered for an additional 10 minutes. Strain and drink. To use as a gargle, add 1/2 teaspoon honey to two ounces of tea. Gargle three times or until mixture is finished. It is okay to swallow this gargle.

Note: Bayberry has high tannin content. Most herbalists recommend it be taken with a small amount of milk to counteract the tannins. Large doses can cause nausea or vomiting.

Bistort Root

Bistort Root is an extremely strong astringent. It is excellent when used as a gargle with respect to inflammation of the mouth and to soothe a sore throat. This may be done several times a day. It can be used in powder form and snorted for clearing the nasal passages. When used as a mouthwash, it will alleviate the symptoms of a sore mouth, swollen or bleeding gums, and canker sores. Simply rub a small amount of fresh powder about the size of a dime on and around your gums and let sit for 30 seconds before rinsing and spitting out. You can continue this process until the sores or swelling are gone. If you have been pushing your voice and find some bleeding or hemorrhaging has occurred in your throat, Bistort root is one of the best herbs for treating this ailment. For Bistort Root tea, bring one pint of water to a boil. Add two tablespoons of fresh powder and let boil for three minutes. Take off heat and let sit for 10 minutes. Strain and let cool until warm enough to drink. You can also take two ounces of tea and mix it with honey for a gargle.

Black Cohosh

Black Cohosh is primarily known as an herb for all uterine troubles in women. However, when made into syrup, it is effective for coughs, including whooping cough because it reduces mucus production. When used in a study on Premenstrual Tension Syndrome, Black Cohosh was shown to reduce hypertension due to its sedative effects on the central nervous system. It is also known to have anti-inflammatory properties when used for muscle pain and arthritis. For dosage and usage, make sure you check with a qualified herbalist or doctor.

Note: Most herbalists do not recommend taking Black Cohosh during pregnancy. Due to its potency, it should not be used for more than one week at a time.

Black Walnut

Due to its high tannin content, Black Walnut is useful for internal cleansing, cleaning out parasites in the digestive tract, including intestinal worms. It has been shown to heal and tone inflamed tissues and is good for healing gums, mouth sores, and soothing the throat. It helps restore enamel to teeth and is used as a natural teeth whitener. For whiter teeth, mix a small amount of the powdered herb into your toothpaste each time you brush. It will look like you are brushing with mud! Don't worry; after you rinse, the brownish tint will be gone. Moreover, when gargled, it is valuable as an anti-fungal herb to help stop possible infections in the throat. Black Walnut is also useful in treating candida infections. Candida can be damaging to the body. It can affect the lymph nodes around the throat causing swelling, discomfort, and overproduction of mucus. For internal cleansing of worms and parasites with Black Walnut, consult a qualified herbalist for daily dosage requirements.

Blue Violet

Blue Violet is excellent for relieving severe headaches and head congestion. It is known to clean mucus from the entire body. When taken internally in capsule form, it alleviates coughs, colds, sore throat, bronchitis, asthma, and stimulates the cleaning out of the bowels. When used as a liquid extract gargle and combined with Sage, Hyssop, Marshmallow and Nettle, it can help with mouth and throat infections. It can also be used as a remedy for nervousness or anxiety when combined with Skullcap or nerve root. When used as a tea, Blue Violet purifies the blood. Brew one tablespoon of fresh powder in three cups of boiling water. Take off heat and let sit for 10 minutes, strain and drink. Drink up to three cups a day for three to four days for severe congestion.

Borage

Borage is good when used as a gargle for mouth and throat sores as well as for loosening phlegm and bringing down swelling in the throat. It is helpful in reducing fevers and lung problems when used as a tea. Borage has been called the "Tea of Courage" because of the calming effect it has on the body and mind, allowing the user to be less nervous or anxious. It is fantastic for calming the entire nervous system. If you have trouble going to sleep, a cup of Borage tea before bed can provide a restful sleep with no grogginess or "feeling out of it" in the morning. Be careful; Borage is very strong. Try small amounts at first to see how your body reacts. Borage may be purchased in bulk leaf form or in a liquid dropper. When using the fresh herb as a tea, bring two cups of water to boil. Add one tablespoon of fresh herb. Let boil for three minutes. Take off heat and let sit covered for 10 minutes. Strain and drink warm.

Brigham Tea

Brigham tea is great for sinus problems and congestion. It acts as a stimulant to the sympathetic nervous system and has a stimulating effect on the bronchial system enabling one to breathe deeper. It is also excellent for allergy conditions. Most studies have shown Brigham tea to contain ephedrine (ephedrine is similar to adrenaline), which may account for its ability to dilate the bronchial passages. Due to this property, it has been used effectively for bronchial asthma. It has also been used effectively in place of caffeine, as well as for depression. However, it may cause nervousness or restlessness in some people, and when used in large doses should be prescribed by a qualified herbal practitioner. To use Brigham tea for the first time, try a small amount in the beginning. Take two medium sized pinches of raw herb (about the size of a golf ball) and boil it in one pint of water for three to five minutes. Remove from heat and let steep covered for 10 minutes. Strain and drink. You may wish to add honey due to its slightly bitter taste.

Bugleweed

Bugleweed is excellent for difficult coughs because of its sedative and narcotic-like properties. Bugleweed can be very calming to the nerves due to its vasoconstrictor actions. To get the most out of this herb, finely cut 1/2 to 1 ounce of the fresh herb, or use two tablespoons of powdered herb. Boil in one pint of water three to five minutes. Remove from heat, strain and let cool. Drink one cup at a time, several times a day as needed. If using the extract, start with 10 drops to see how your body reacts. If need be you can increase the drops, but do not exceed more than 30 drops at one time.

Note: Most herbalists do not recommend long term use due to a potential decrease in thyroid function.

Burdock

Burdock is one of the best blood purifiers known in the herbal kingdom. It is extremely useful to help heal a sore throat because of its high levels of antibacterials and antifungals. This herb is often used by herbalists to resolve liver congestion. Eating Burdock has a slight cleansing effect on the bowels, which is good for removing unwanted mucus from the body that could find its way into the throat. Ancient herbalists believed that Burdock had magical qualities and used it to keep away negative spirits. When a sore throat or cold is coming on or is present, two capsules three times a day is very effective. To drink as a tea, add two tablespoons of fresh herb to one pint of boiling water, cover and boil for three to five minutes. Take off heat and let sit covered for 10 minutes. Strain and drink warm. Add honey to taste.

Calamint

Calamint is a wonderful herb to use when experiencing attacks of asthma or bronchitis because of its expectorant qualities. It is a member of the mint family, and almost all herbs in this family are good for digestion as well. It may be used to help calm the nerves and aid in easing joint pain due to arthritis and rheumatism. Calamint is helpful when you are experiencing chest congestion and having trouble breathing. Throughout the day and before bed, rub the size of a quarter of Calamint oil on your chest and lower neck. You may also apply the oil to the bottom of your feet; this works by the oil being absorbed through your feet into your body. Rub the oil on your shoulders and neck after strenuous performances if you have strained your neck or throat while singing.

Catnip

Catnip is generally used as a mood elevator. It is helpful for tension, stress, anxiety, nervousness and insomnia. Many people use Catnip as a natural alternative to over-the-counter sleeping pills. It is very strong and can be used regularly without any feeling of waking up groggy or tired in the morning. Two capsules 30 minutes before bedtime will certainly afford a good nights sleep. When used as a tea, boil one pint of water and then allow the water to simmer down for several minutes. Never boil Catnip as it will render the herb useless. Remove the water from the heat source and add two tablespoons of herb (freshly cut if possible) or one tablespoon of powder. Let steep covered for 10 minutes, strain and drink. Catnip is not the tastiest herb when used as a tea, and honey may be added to make it more palatable. If you do not have the fresh herb, you may add 1/2 dropper of liquid extract to a cup of warm water and drink 20 minutes before bedtime.

Cayenne

Cayenne is also known as Capsicum. It is one of the most useful herbs around, and enough cannot be said about its miraculous healing properties. It is extremely stimulating to the entire body. When used in moderation, it causes no harm and has no unhealthy reactions. Cayenne is outstanding for digestion as an aid in cleaning the colon and intestinal walls. It is excellent for all throat infections or swollen cords. Cayenne has been shown to work well with vitamin C. Some herbalists feel this is because Cayenne helps improve the absorption of Vitamin C into the bloodstream. Cayenne is incomparable in its use for circulation and keeping one warm in cold temperatures. Take two to four capsules in the morning and in the afternoon. Sprinkled on your meals, it will greatly aid your digestion, helping you to better absorb your food. If you have to sing during the winter months when it is very cold and your voice feels stiff due to the temperature, sprinkle a pinch or two of Cayenne powder into your shoes. Shake it around so it covers the entire shoe and then wear your shoes as you regularly would. The herb will absorb through your feet as your feet begin to sweat, allowing it to enter into your bloodstream. Be sure you only start with a small pinch or two. If you use too much, you will actually begin to taste cayenne throughout the day. To reduce a sore throat, stop inflammation, and stop potential infection, gargle with Cayenne powder. Add a small pinch of Cayenne powder and a tablespoon of honey to two ounces of warm water. Mix well and gargle until the mixture is gone. Cayenne is one of the main herbs in Superior Vocal Health's "Vocal Rescue" Gargle.

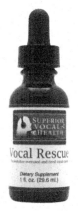

Note: Cayenne will color your socks and shoes when it meets with the perspiration of your feet. Black socks may be best for this use.

Chamomile

Best known in the West for its soothing qualities, Chamomile is actually a stimulant with antispasmodic properties. It is excellent for a number of ailments including bronchitis, colds, allergies, and headaches due to tension and stress. It has a calming effect on the entire body. While not as powerful as some of the other herbs such as Valerian, Skullcap, or Lobelia, it is good for soothing the stomach and for mild nervousness. Chamomile can be taken and used effectively in almost any form of tea, powder, capsule, or crushed plant. For a good allergy season remedy, drink three to four cups of Chamomile throughout the day. You can find Chamomile in tea bag form at any health food store. For additional allergy relief, you can also put brewed Chamomile tea into a Neti Pot for a sinus flush (see Neti Pot section) as well as in a steamer to inhale the fumes.

Chickweed

Chickweed is known to have demulcent properties and to heal and soothe almost anything. It is high in Vitamin C. It is excellent when used for hoarseness, coughs, colds, inflammation in the throat, lungs, and bronchial passages, and for swollen or inflamed vocal cords and throat muscles. It is also a blood purifier. It liquefies and removes mucus from the entire respiratory tract. This is important because when the respiratory tract fills with too much mucus, it begins to clog our system not allowing the lungs to function as they should and limiting access to our breath, vocal chamber and resonance. To use as a tea, brew two tablespoons of fresh herb in one pint of boiling water. Brew for three to five minutes, take off heat and let sit covered for 15 minutes. Strain and drink warm. Drink two to four cups a day until mucus is gone.

Chlorophyll

Chlorophyll is the pigment found in green plants which contains enzymes that help decompose superoxide radicals in the body into a more manageable form. This has been shown to help slow down the aging process. It helps rebuild and replenish our red blood cells, boost our energy, and increase our well being. It is an effective gargle for healing and soothing a sore throat. It is also an excellent remedy for bad breath. Chlorophyll is an anti-inflammatory and can be taken every day either in raw form or through various green food sources, especially Wheatgrass, Spirulina and Chlorella. If you feel a sore throat coming on, immediately gargle with one ounce of Wheatgrass or pure Chlorophyll liquid. Use a 1/2 ounce at a time for a total of two gargles. Swallow the juice after you gargle. To super-charge your chlorophyll gargle, add a pinch of cayenne to the juice.

Cinnamon

Some herbalists rely on Cinnamon for complete body healing and recommend it for daily use. It is superb for healing and soothing sore throats as well as eliminating excess flatulence. Cinnamon has been used for thousands of years and is referenced as an herb Moses used when mixing oils for anointing. It is very useful when taken as a tea to induce sweating and to break up mucus, fever, and congestion. When preparing a tea, if possible use fresh sticks and cloves. Add two sticks of the herb to three cups of water and boil covered for three to five minutes. Let steep for 20 minutes. Add honey and some lemon for taste and a more powerful healing effect.

Collinsonia

Collinsonia soothes the mucus membranes. It has slight astringent properties and relieves inflammation of the throat due to colds and flu. Congestion, irritation, constriction, chronic laryngitis, pharyngitis, and some forms of chronic bronchitis respond very well to Collinsonia due to its ability to release and open up constricted areas. It mends voices experiencing fatigue from speaking and pressing on the cords. It releases throat constriction and allows more blood to flow through the inflamed and constricted overused areas. Collinsonia helps to stabilize the lining of the sinus cavities and minimize buildup of excess mucus in various parts of the body including the sinus cavities and throat. To use as a gargle, mix one full dropper of liquid extract in two ounces of warm water, gargle for 30 seconds, then swallow.

Swallowing Collinsonia stimulates your digestive system and is helpful in treating irritable bowel syndrome. If you are brave enough, you may also put five to ten drops of liquid extract in a Neti Pot and use as directed. It is very strong, so be prepared!

Coltsfoot

The botanical name for Coltsfoot, Tussilago, translates into "cough dispeller." Coltsfoot has traditionally been used to treat coughs, whooping cough, asthma, excess mucus, bronchitis, and laryngitis. The flowers and leaves of Coltsfoot are used for their demulcent and expectorant properties. I would not recommend it, but in Europe a remedy for asthma and some other bronchial disorders is smoking Coltsfoot along with a few other similar acting herbs. To make a tea of Clotsfoot, add three tablespoons of herb to one pint of boiling water. Boil for three to five minutes. Take off heat and let sit covered for 15 minutes. Strain and drink warm, up to three glasses per day for up to three days. Drink this tea if you are experiencing severe cases of asthmatic congestion, bronchitis, or allergies. Coltsfoot has a slightly bitter taste, so add honey or other sweetener as needed.

> **Note:** Both Coltsfoot and Comfrey contains a group of compounds called pyrrolizidine alkaloids. When used over a long period of time (more than two weeks) it can be toxic to the liver; therefore, most herbalists recommend only short term use.

Comfrey

Comfrey has traditionally been used for the healing of fractures and bruises. Because of its general soothing effect and ability to clear the mucus membranes, it is often used to treat difficult coughs, hoarseness, sore throat, and respiratory issues. Because of its demulcent properties, it soothes and coats the throat lining. Comfrey is also high in potassium, thereby providing the body with natural energy. Add one full dropper of liquid extract of Comfrey to two cups of boiling water. Take off heat and let sit for five minutes, then drink. Drink two times per day for up to three days.

Note: Both Comfrey and Coltsfoot contain a group of compounds called pyrrolizidine alkaloids. When used over a long period of time (more than two weeks) it can be toxic to the liver; therefore, most herbalists recommend only short term use.

Echinacea

Echinacea is considered one of nature's most useful herbs. It is most commonly used as a cleansing herb and purifier. It can work wonders for a sore throat or any mouth, gum, or throat issue when applied directly to the affected area or when used as a gargle. When combined with Myrrh, it is extremely effective for all throat issues. (See Specific Herbal Formula section.) Echinacea has such powerful antibiotic effects that it is often prescribed as an ongoing remedy to boost and support the immune system by helping to rid the body of toxins. It may be taken on a regular basis without any adverse effects. If you feel symptoms of sickness coming on, begin taking a full dropper of liquid extract in a recommended tea (see cold formula section) or two capsules of Echinacea three times a day. Echinacea can be found in all the current herbal formulas from Superior Vocal Health.

Elderberry

Native Americans used Elderberry to reduce fever and relieve aching joints. It helps with inflammation by relieving coughs and congestion. It can be used for allergies when using the aerial parts of the plant for tea. It cleanses the system, enhances immunity, soothes the respiratory tract, and helps break up mucus. Certain compounds in Elderberry bind with viruses before they can penetrate the walls of cells, thereby inhibiting their ability to spread. Some evidence suggests that chemicals in Elder flower and berries may help reduce swelling of mucous membranes in the sinuses, helping to relieve nasal congestion. To make a tea, brew two teaspoonfuls of fresh herb in one pint of covered boiling water for three to five minutes. Take off heat and let sit covered for 15 minutes, strain and drink. Drink three cups throughout the day for up to one week.

Elecampane

Elecampane has expectorant, antiseptic, and astringent properties. It is superb for chest and bronchial ailments, especially when combined with Echinacea, because it restores and invigorates the respiratory system. It warms and strengthens the lungs and promotes expectoration. It strengthens, cleanses, and tones the mucus membranes of the lungs and stomach. At the first sign of a respiratory issue, taking Elecampane may highly reduce the time and severity of the issue. Two capsules three times per day with food works very well. When you feel congested, use one full dropper of liquid extract of Elecampane with Echinacea in a cup of hot water. Let sit for five minutes, then drink. Continue drinking this tea until you feel relief of symptoms. Add honey for taste.

Eucalyptus

The oil of Eucalyptus is is one of the best natural antiseptic oils known in the herbal kingdom. It is effective when used for hay fever, allergies, coughs, colds, and chronic respiratory mucus overproduction. It can open up the sinus passages and lungs due to colds and bronchial maladies. One of its oils, Eucalyptol, has been found to be an expectorant, decongestant, reliever of coughs, and killer of bacteria. It produces excellent results when the oil is inhaled through a Neti Pot (see Neti Pot section) or in a steam. If you are having serious congestion in your sinuses, see the "What do I do When" section for a powerful remedy.

Fenugreek

Fenugreek is great for relieving a sore throat and will also help clear mucus from the bronchial and sinus passages. It aids in reducing inflammation and swelling. It is also known to decrease appetite. Fenugreek has some properties that resemble estrogen, which explain its use in helping a slow sex drive and adding vibrancy and energy to one's system. The seeds of Fenugreek are useful for acid reflux and heartburn. They contain a high level of mucilage which helps the digestive system by coating the lining of the stomach and intestines, decreasing inflammation. If you suffer from acid reflux or heartburn, sprinkle a tablespoon of ground seeds onto your salad or meal. To make a tea, brew two teaspoonfuls of fresh herb in one pint of covered boiling water for three to five minutes. Take off heat and let sit covered for 15 minutes, strain and drink.

Note: Most herbalists do not recommend using Fenugreek during pregnancy as it has the ability to induce labor.

Feverfew

Feverfew has been called a "wonder herb" when used for intense headaches. It is a safe, natural alternative to aspirin. Aspirin thins the blood and can be dangerous to a singer, causing rupture of the veins that feed the cords their blood supply. Feverfew is used for treating colds, fevers, flu, and allergies. It can relieve gas and bloating as well as help remove parasites and intestinal worms. To make a tea, brew two teaspoonfuls of fresh herb in one pint of covered boiling water for three to five minutes. Take off heat and let sit covered for 10 minutes, strain and drink.

Note: Feverfew may promote the onset of a woman's menstrual cycle. Most herbalists do not recommend using it during pregnancy.

Flaxseed

Flaxseed is a well-known herb, especially the oil derived from the seed. It is used for coughs and asthma. Because of its amazing health benefits, some herbalists believe Flaxseed to be one of the most important individual herbs a person can take. Flaxseed is high in protein and fiber and helps every part of the body function better, including the cardiovascular, immune and nervous systems. If you are constipated due to travel that includes flying or eating poorly on the road, mix two to three tablespoons of Flaxseed oil into a cup of juice three times a day, and drink. This will keep you clean and free of debris and eliminate constipation. If you do not like the taste, carry capsules with you. Take two to three capsules in the same fashion. Make sure you put the Flaxseed oil and/or capsules under refrigeration. By staying clean, you will feel lighter, more energetic, and more focused when you need to sing or speak.

Garlic

Garlic is one of the most powerful herbs known for fighting infection, especially when it comes to infections of the throat. Garlic is a natural antibiotic; however, it does not destroy the body's natural flora in the intestine and colon. In fact, it is praised for its digestion benefits. It is a serious immune booster. When used as a detoxifier, garlic rejuvenates the entire system and purges the body of unwanted debris. If you feel some type of sickness or sore throat coming on, chop up one or two cloves of garlic into small pieces. Chew the pieces slowly until they are like liquid. Make sure you chew thoroughly, allowing the juice to coat and sit in your throat and mouth for at least two minutes then swallow. Chewing is very important because the antibiotic healing element in garlic, allicin, is only activated when it is crushed. Once allicin enters the stomach, it begins to heal your entire body. Chewing garlic may stop the infection altogether or stop it from getting worse. Garlic is one of the main herbs in Sinus Clear Out from Superior Vocal Health.

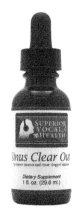

Note: Garlic can leave a strong odor on your breath. Chew Parsley to minimize bad breath.

Ginger

Ginger is most commonly used in aiding digestion by helping to expel excess mucus from the body. When taken during the cold winter months, it warms the entire body. Ginger is highly recommended when traveling because it keeps the digestive system regular. It is also a great herb for acid reflux. Ginger helps the throat to stay wet and promotes saliva when chewed raw. When you must sing and are experiencing tired, overused cords or have dry mouth due to nervousness, chew a small piece of Ginger about the size and thickness of a quarter five minutes before you sing. This will get the saliva flowing and stimulate your entire throat and vocal mechanism. Ginger is also excellent to drink as a tea on a regular basis, especially

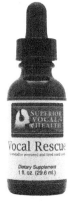

during the colder months when the body needs to be warm and energized for singing. Every voice professional should carry Ginger tea bags with them at all times. Ginger is one of the main herbs in the Vocal Rescue formula from Superior Vocal Health.

Gingko Biloba

Gingko Biloba is a widely used herb in Chinese Medicine for slow or imbalanced circulation. It is effective in improving blood circulation to the heart and brain and keeping the mind clear, energized, and alert. It also relieves bronchial constriction due to asthma and is commonly prescribed for treating a low sex drive. Ginko is often combined with Ginseng to help with low energy and conditions related to cold weather such as coldness in the organs and blood circulation. Take Ginko before singing to provide energy to the whole body without the side effects that come along with caffeine consumption. Ginko has been shown to help improve memory, an added plus when needing to recall lyrics or lines or notes for presentations. Two capsules in the morning with food is a good dose for memory and alertness. One full dropper of liquid extract in a cup of Ginger or Green tea is also effective in waking up the whole body.

> **Note:** Most herbalists recommend that anyone taking prescription blood-thinning medication or over-the-counter pain killers consult a physician before taking Ginko Bilboa.

Ginseng

Worldwide, there are up to 22 different plants and at least 10 different species of Ginseng. Panax Ginseng refers to American and Asian Ginseng. Its name is derived from the Greek word "panacea" or "cure all." Siberian Ginseng is also part of the Ginseng family but not genus as pure Ginseng. Ginseng is considered an adaptogen and has been used in China for thousands of years to treat many different kinds of illnesses. It promotes healthy lung function and aids lack of energy. American Ginseng is used by athletes for overall body strengthening. It is very effective in warming the entire body and can produce perspiration. It can be used as a tea for sore throat, cough, and chest troubles. It is useful for helping to keep the mind clear and focused, and in bolstering the immune system. American Ginseng is more sought after in Asia due to its different qualities than Asian Ginseng. American Ginseng tends to have a sweeter taste, and its healing properties are used to cool, nourishing the Yin or cooler temperament. Asian Ginseng has the opposite effect and stimulates, nourishing the Yang or warmer temperament. Ginseng tea can be found in any health food store in tea bag form. If taking it in tea form, two cups a day using a tea bag per cup is good for overall body health and energy. If taking capsules, two in the morning and one more mid-day will provide extra energy. Ginseng extract is as effective as tea bags and capsules. Use one full dropper in a cup of green or Ginger tea. Add honey to taste.

> **Note:** American Ginseng has shown in numerous studies that it does not have an adverse effect on those with high blood pressure. However, these studies were not done with Panax and Siberian Ginseng. Therefore, most herbalists do not recommend taking Siberian or Panax Ginseng if you have high blood pressure, as it may cause excitability and nervous tension.

Goldenseal
Goldenseal has been called a "miracle herb" because of its total healing effect. Powder or extract is generally considered to be more effective than tea. For upper respiratory infections, it should be used when infection has already set in and the mucus is yellow or greenish. Goldenseal is very effective when used for tonsillitis and other difficult throat troubles. It may be used as a gargle (five drops of extract in two ounces of warm water). It may also be taken internally for digestion difficulties or infection in the sinus passages and respiratory tract. For superior herbal healing formulas that use Goldenseal, see the Specific Herbal Formulas section of this book.

> **Note:** Most herbalists do not recommend taking Goldenseal for more than a week at a time because it can reduce the absorption of the B vitamins. If you do take Goldenseal, it is recommended to

allow at least two weeks in between dosages. Do not use if pregnant, as it may stimulate the uterus. If you experience diarrhea and nausea, stop taking immediately. If you have any heart disease or hypertension, do not take Goldenseal as it can stimulate the heart muscle thus increasing blood pressure.

Gotu Cola

Gotu Cola is often referred to as the "memory herb" because it has been shown to stimulate the nervous system, aiding in blood circulation to the brain and helping to relieve mental fatigue. In Ayurvedic medicine, this herb is one of the most important herbs used. Long ago in Sri Lanka, elephants were seen eating large amounts of Gotu Cola on a regular basis as a standard part of their diet. Elephants are notorious for their excellent memory and longevity. Because of its effect on the brain, it is also used to aid those with slight depression. One capsule in the morning and one in the afternoon is a good dose to start with. For extra support during rehearsals or a performance, add one dropperful of extract to a cup of Green Tea and drink 20 minutes before working.

Green Tea

Green Tea is well known for its potential protection against heart disease, ulcers, and cancer. It has antibacterial and antioxidant properties. Green Tea does contain caffeine, but only about half the amount of a cup of coffee. Due to this smaller content, it has a good effect on relieving headaches. Another added benefit of Green Tea is its high levels of theanine. Theanine is an amino acid that helps calm the mind and improve mental focus without leaving you feeling drowsy or foggy. It is an excellent tea to drink before performing or rehearsals because of the small lift of energy and the added effect of the theanine. For an excellent energy formula to drink before singing, see the Specific Herbal Formula section under "Energy and Endurance Formulas."

Grindelia

Grindelia, also known as Gumweed, is used for its expectorant and mild sedative properties and easing dry hacking coughs. It is listed in the United States Pharmacopoeia as an internal remedy for asthma, bronchitis, and other upper respiratory tract ailments. A preparation of Grindelia can be used to bring a relaxing effect on the muscles lining the smaller bronchial passages. This aids in clearing mucus in the respiratory passages.

> **Note:** Some people have found that using high doses of Grindelia can be toxic. In addition, it may cause irritation in the kidneys or stomach. It should only be used when administered by a competent herbal practitioner.

Hawthorn

Hawthorn extract of leaves and flowers has an antispasmodic effect on the body and may be used for stress relief and insomnia. It helps in calming mental agitation, decreasing restlessness, and reducing nervous palpitations. It has a strengthening action on the heart which also helps many problems related to blood pressure. It opens up the arteries, promoting circulation and improving the blood supply to all the tissues in the body. Hawthorn is an excellent choice for those singing or performing in cold climates to help keep the body warm and energy flowing to the chest and lungs. If you feel the need to relax or settle down before singing, add one tablespoon of Hawthorn, Chamomile, and Hops to one pint of boiling water. Boil covered for three to five minutes. Steep covered for 20 minutes. Strain and drink hot. You can store this tea in the refrigerator for up to one week and take it with you, using it as needed. If you are using extracts, start with 10 drops of each in a cup of warm water. Add more as needed.

Hops

Hops is a well known herb used for insomnia, nerves, anxiousness, and over abundance of sexual energy because it relaxes the entire nervous system. Hops also has antibiotic properties that help speed recovery when healing from staph infections. If you are experiencing insomnia, take a handful of fresh hops flowers and stuff your pillow before going to bed. Then have a cup of hops tea. This is said to give one a very restful sleep.

> **Note:** Most herbalists recommend that Hops should not be used by people who take antidepressant medication.

Horehound

Horehound is an all around remedy herb that should be kept on hand for regular use. It is one of the most widely used herbs for relieving difficult and pressing coughs. Syrup made from Horehound is excellent for chronic sore throats, colds, asthma, and difficulty breathing. It is a gentle expectorant and loosens phlegm from the chest. It will sustain the vocal cords during congestion and hoarseness. A strong cup of Horehound tea has the ability to loosen phlegm impacted in the throat and sinus passages. For a tonic for the respiratory organs, bring one pint of water to a boil and add two tablespoons of the fresh herb. Boil covered for three to five minutes. Remove from heat and steep covered for 20 minutes. Strain and drink while still warm. Drink two cups a day for three days. You may want to add some honey for taste.

> **Note:** Herbalists have noted that larger doses of Horehound may cause irregular heart rhythm. It has been suggested to not be taken when pregnant.

Horseradish

Horseradish root is well known for its cleansing properties. Raw, fresh Horseradish can open up the worst clogged sinus passages. It is also excellent for those with poor or low blood circulation, warming the whole body especially in the winter months. Its ability to induce perspiration 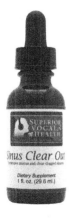 makes it a useful herb to break up cold and flu symptoms while warming the chest and lungs. In addition, it is an excellent aid for the digestive system, as it stimulates the secretion of gastric juices. When experiencing severe clogged sinuses, some people have been known to rub a small amount of horseradish about the size of a dime between their eyes just above the nose. If you are brave enough to try this, start with a small amount and be careful not to get the herb in your eyes. For a warming winter tea to open the chest and throat before singing, bring one pint of water to a boil. Add one tablespoon of Horseradish, Ginger and 1/2 tablespoon of Ginseng. Boil covered for three minutes. Remove from heat and let sit covered for 20 minutes. Strain and drink as needed. Horseradish is one of the herbs in Sinus Clear Out from Superior Vocal Health.

> **Note:** When preparing Horseradish, keep away from the eyes and avoid excessive contact with the skin. Most herbalists recommended that people with thyroid conditions should not use Horseradish because it contains compounds that can impede the production of hormones by the thyroid gland.

Hyssop

Hyssop is referred to in the Bible as a healing herb. It is mentioned in Psalm 51:7: "Purge me with Hyssop and I shall be clean; wash me and I shall be whiter than snow." Along with Sage, it was also used in Biblical times to clean out sacred spaces. It is used by herbalists for pulmonary conditions such as asthma, colds, coughs, and all lung disorders. It works very well in loosening phlegm from the throat and lungs, as well as the mucus lining of the stomach. See the Specific Herbal Formulas section for tired and overused voices to find an excellent formula for a sore throat using Hyssop.

> **Note:** Most herbalists recommend not using Hyssop for more than two weeks straight. In addition it is not advised for use by pregnant women due to its capacity to stimulate menstruation.

Jaborandi

Jaborandi is an herb found in the Amazon forest. When translated it means "slobber weed" because of its amazing ability to increase salivation in large levels. Jaborandi is used for breaking up colds and is also effective for respiratory illnesses such as asthma. In addition, it has been used, but not tested clinically, for baldness by natives in the Amazon and to help alleviate the symptoms of glaucoma. For help with dry mouth issues, brew an ounce of fresh leaves in a pint of covered boiling water for 20 minutes. Take off heat and let sit for 10 minutes. Strain and drink warm or cold 10 minutes before singing or speaking.

Kava Kava

Kava Kava is excellent for insomnia, anxiety, stress and headaches without having the side effects and addictive potential of narcotics like Valium and Xanax. Although not its primary use, it has also worked for respiratory issues such as asthma. This may be due to its calming effect, allowing a person to breathe more freely when the body is in a higher state of relaxation. Natives on some Pacific Islands consume Kava in large doses to reach a euphoric state that causes them to have hallucinations; however this is not recommended.

Note: Consult a competent herbal practitioner before using Kava Kava. It should not be used with alcohol. Most herbalists do not recommend Kava Kava for people under the age of 18, pregnant women, nursing mothers, or those who suffer from depression or take anti-anxiety drugs.

Lemon Balm

Lemon Balm has been used as an herbal remedy for nervousness, anxiety, and relaxation for more than 2000 years. In Medieval times, it was a very popular drink. Concoctions of Lemon Balm were made up and mixed with wine to cure fevers and lift the spirits. Many Arab countries attribute this herb to creating increased intelligence in those who take it daily. Its essential oil is commonly used by massage therapists to relax their patients. Today, most herbalists use Lemon Balm or its essential oil as a calming agent for nerves, anxiety, depression, and sleep disorders, as well as to strengthen the memory and mind. In Germany, Lemon Balm is a common prescription allowed by the government for insomnia due to nervous conditions. It is also excellent at removing mucus in cases of acute bronchitis, due to its ability to relax the respiratory system allowing it to drain more effectively. For a very relaxing tea, put three tablespoons of crushed herb into one pint of boiling water. Boil covered for two to three minutes, then steep covered for 15 minutes. Strain and drink 20 minutes before bedtime or when you want to relax. This will relax you without the side effects of prescription drugs.

Licorice
Licorice is a wonderful herb that helps treat many different ailments such as stomach ulcers, colitis, headaches, and respiratory ailments because of its high levels of glycyrrhizin. Glycyrrhizin is a natural sweetener that is 50 times sweeter than sugar. Licorice has expectorant and demulcent properties and is most effective when used for congestion and bronchitis. It helps to heal inflamed tissues and membranes due to its anti-inflammatory and anti-allergic properties. It has been used successfully for sore throat and injured throat muscles, but it does have a mild laxative effect when taken in high doses. Some people confuse licorice candy with Licorice herb. The former has little or no Licorice herb in it at all. Licorice candy has Anise oil in it, which tastes very much like Licorice but does not heal the same as Licorice herb. If you suck on Licorice candy when trying to heal a sore throat, it will have little or no effect. Licorice is also used to purge the liver and body of unwanted debris when taken as a cleansing agent. To help heal an overused and tired voice using Licorice, see the Specific Herbal Formulas section.

Note: Side effects of Licorice can be very dangerous when used improperly. Always consult a qualified herbal practitioner before using it internally in high doses. It is not recommended for people with high blood pressure, heart disease, diabetes, severe menstrual problems, history of stroke. or by pregnant women. In addition it is not recommended for use on a daily basis, as it has been known to cause high blood pressure.

Marshmallow
Marshmallow is used for hoarseness, coughs, and lung trouble including bronchitis. It exudes a sweet mucilage that is soothing, softening, and healing. It aids the body in expelling excess fluid and mucus by soothing and healing the mucus membranes. Marshmallow has been prescribed for centuries as the herb traditionally taken to soothe inflammation and irritation in the digestive system (acting as a slight laxative) as well as in the respiratory and urinary tracts. Syrup and lozenges made from Marshmallow are excellent for coughs. Gargling with Marshmallow can alleviate mouth sores and swollen or

inflamed gums. It is extremely effective when combined with other soothing herbs for a sore throat or overused voice. See the Specific Herbal Formulas section to get the most out of Marshmallow.

Mullein

Mullein can be used as a gargle for a sore throat and for tonsillitis when the tonsils are swollen and inflamed. Syrup from Mullein has been used for centuries to help reduce nasty coughs. It is useful for asthma, bronchitis, and difficulty breathing brought on by asthma. A tea made from the flowers is known to induce sleep because of its sedative properties, as well as pain relief due to its narcotic properties. In larger doses, it may act as a laxative. For relief from a persistent cough and chest congestion, brew one tablespoon of fresh herb in three cups of covered boiling water for three to five minutes. Remove from heat and let steep covered for 10 minutes. Strain and drink. Drink two cups a day for one week.

> **Note:** When straining, make sure to strain the concoction through a fine cloth to remove any plant hairs that could irritate the throat and digestive tract.

Myrrh

Myrrh is another herb commonly used and found in the Bible. It is useful because of its astringent effect which causes contraction of body tissues and its antiseptic properties which are effective against viral infections. It is a stimulant and tonic for bronchial and lung problems because it diminishes mucus discharge. Myrrh also helps with blood circulation and can aid in keeping you warm while singing. When taken internally in capsule form, it can help reduce halitosis or bad breath. In Ayurvedic medicine, Myrrh is used regularly as a remedy for sore throat, gum disease and mouth sores. In Germany, the government has allowed Myrrh to be prescribed by doctors as treatment for mild inflammation of the mouth and throat. If you are experiencing difficulty with sore gums, take a small amount of fresh Myrrh powder about the size of a dime and put it on your toothbrush. Add a touch of water to make it into a slight paste. Brush your gums thoroughly with the paste for at least one full minute. Rinse out afterwards. Do this twice a day for five to seven days and you will see your gums fast on their way to being healed and normal again. If you cannot find powdered herb, this procedure may also be done with a full dropper of liquid extract in an ounce of water swished around the gums for two minutes.

Nettle

When used in tea form, Nettle will expel phlegm from the lungs and stomach, as well as clean out the urinary passages. It has been used for centuries as one of the standard herbs to deal with and heal asthma and other bronchial issues by cleansing and detoxifying the entire body of unwanted waste. Nettle is very high in potassium, iron, and silica, making it an excellent herb for overall body health and recovery when one has been sick for some time. According to some traditions, when fighting in the colder climates the Roman soldiers used Nettle leaves to keep their legs warm. Nettle can be used to battle allergies affecting the voice and throat. For an excellent remedy during allergy season and also to combat hay fever, mix two full droppers of Nettle liquid extract and 1/2 dropper of Echinacea in two ounces of juice. Drink three times a day for up to five days.

Nerve Root

Nerve root, also called Lady's Slipper or American Valerian, was commonly used by Native Americans to calm the nerves and sooth the soul. It has antispasmodic properties and is often used to alleviate depression and elevate the mood. It has the same effect as Valerian, but not as strong. The good thing about Nerve Root is that it does not have narcotic properties, which can be helpful for people with addictive tendencies. The active ingredients of Nerve Root are not water soluble, so it is best taken in liquid extract form. Nerve Root can also be used for insomnia and anxiety when mixed properly with other similar affecting herbs such as Skullcap and Catnip. If you have trouble sleeping the night before performances, presentations and auditions, take Nerve Root 30 minutes before going to bed. This can provide you with a deep, restful sleep and you will not wake up feeling groggy or tired like one does from over-the-counter sleeping pills.

Note: Most herbalists do not recommend taking Nerve Root in large doses (more than 10 drops) or for more than three days at a time, as it may cause hallucinations.

Oil of Oregano

Oil of Oregano is one of the most powerful remedies for viral infections, stomach poisons, bronchial and respiratory ailments, colds and flu. It has been thoroughly tested and proven to have antibacterial, antiviral, antiparasitic, antiseptic, and antifungal properties. However, this is not the Oregano oil you use in your kitchen. This is wild grown Mediterranean Oregano oil. Tests comparing oil of Oregano to antibiotics have shown it to be as or more effective in fighting infection because our body does not become resistant to oil of Oregano like it can when continually taking antibiotics. It is also outstanding for supporting the immune system. This miracle herb can be used for an endless list of ailments from herpes and candida to throat and chest infections or fighting infectious disease. No singer or voice professional should be without oil of Oregano. The moment I feel any kind of respiratory issue or even the slightest cough creeping in, I immediately begin taking oil of Oregano. Within days, I am healed from what could have been a two or three week disaster. If you feel sickness coming on, put two or three drops into four ounces of juice, three times per day. Continue for at least one week to make sure you are getting enough of the oil into your system. The oil is very potent and may be too powerful or difficult to handle due to the sting it can cause in the throat. If this is the case, you can purchase empty pill capsules online or at any health food store. Open the capsule and drop four to eight drops into the capsule, then close it back up. Take one capsule three times a day for a week. If you find you still have a small amount of respiratory difficulty after one week, continue the dosage for another week. Make sure you take the capsule immediately after you drop the oil into it; if you do not, within a few minutes the capsule will begin to melt.

Note: With all the positive attention in the press and medical fields about the extraordinary healing properties of oil of Oregano, many companies have begun to put out diluted and ill prepared products. The agent in Oregano oil that is responsible for its incredible healing abilities is called carvacrol. Make sure that any product you buy has a carvacrol level of at least 60% and is mixed with organic virgin olive oil. Otherwise you are getting a diluted and potentially unhealthy mixture.

Origanum

Origanum, also called European Oregano, is given by many herbal practitioners to women to help with menstrual difficulties. It is also effective when used as a gargle for a sore throat and can be used for tonsillitis, bronchitis, asthma, coughs, and other respiratory issues. In addition, it is useful when applied as a healing compress for a sore throat due to excessive stress or overused, tired muscles after a performance. For a healing compress, steep two large tablespoons of herb in 1/2 pint of boiling water for 30 minutes. Take a small clean cotton towel large enough to wrap around your neck and let it soak in the solution for 20 minutes. After soaking it, wring out the towel, but not so much that you lose the concentration of the formula in the towel. Wrap the warm (not too hot) towel around your neck for 10 minutes or until it becomes cool. You can keep your neck warm and the heat in the towel longer as well as avoid excess drip from the liquid by wearing a scarf around the wrap. Soak the cloth again for five minutes in the solution and use as a wrap for another 10 minutes.

Osha

Osha is an antibacterial herb with similar properties found in Echinacea. However, Osha works more effectively on the lungs, helping to reduce and expel unwanted phlegm due to infection, colds, and flu. It is excellent for warding off viral infection in the sinuses and throat. Many natural cough syrups are made with Osha as the primary ingredient. Native American Indians in Arizona have used Osha to help cure sore throats, common colds, cough, and sinusitis.

For a very effective chest cold remedy using Osha, see the Specific Herbal Formulas section below.

Parsley

Parsley is well known for its use in cooking. It is an excellent source of vitamins A, B1, B2, C and iron. Traditionally, Parsley has been used for stomach disorders and flatulence. However, it also works to eliminate bad breath, neutralizing foul odor caused by ill digestion or improper food combinations. After singing for some time, most singers experience bad breath due to stress from performance, deep open breathing, and "digging deep" into the diaphragm for support. It can be very embarrassing when accepting praise after a wonderful performance to have unbearable breath. An easy solution to this problem is to dip a few sprigs of Parsley into some organic apple cider vinegar. Put the Parsley into a Ziploc bag or container to store during the performance. After the performance and before meeting your admirers, chew the Parsley for several minutes until it is almost liquid, then swallow. This will help destroy bad breath and make sure your fans keep coming back for more!

> **Note:** Some herbalists do not recommend taking large amounts of Parsley, as it is a uterine stimulant. If you suffer from inflammatory kidney disease, refrain from using large amounts of Parsley.

Passion Flower

Passion Flower is used for its calming, sedative, pain relieving action. Herbalists prescribe it to treat anxiety, insomnia, muscle spasms, stress, headaches, seizures, hysteria and hyperactivity in children. Passion Flower's unique calming quality tones the sympathetic nerves and improves blood circulation and the nutrition that the nerves receive. In the United States, Passion Flower has been banned due to claims that the herb's ability to effectively do what it says it does have gone unproven. However, in Europe it is widely used for all the above issues, particularly as a mild sedative and non-addicting tranquilizer. Passion Flower can be a safe and reliable remedy for performance anxiety and stage fright or insomnia due to nerves the night before performances. For a calming experience, add two tablespoons of

Passion Flower to a pint of boiling water. Reduce heat and let sit covered for 15 minutes. Strain and drink. If you do not have the fresh herb, you may use liquid extract. Add 1/2 dropper of liquid extract of Passion Flower into a warm cup of Chamomile tea. If you need more potency, add as you wish. Try Passion Flower first at a time when you can monitor it is effects, such as before a rehearsal, so you will know how much to use before an actual performance or presentation.

> **Note:** Most herbalists recommend not taking Passion Flower with MAO (Monoamine Oxidase) inhibiting antidepressants or during pregnancy or lactation, as its safety during these times has not yet been determined.

Peppermint
Peppermint is a wonderful stimulant and a very popular oil for healing with aromatherapy because it contains menthol. However, this is not the same make up as the menthol in cough drops, which is usually mixed with sugar and other chemicals. One of the most common uses of Peppermint is for healing and soothing digestive issues such as intestinal cramping, stomach aches, and excess gas. When used in its raw herb form, a strong cup of pure Peppermint tea will relieve coughs, open the sinuses, and stimulate the body as well as any cup of coffee or tea, without the harmful side effects such as jitters, loss of appetite, and nervousness. You may not feel the results as quickly or intensely as caffeine, because caffeine over-stimulates the system by robbing energy from the nervous system. Peppermint tea instead will support the deeper energy in your system and activate it to evenly support your energy needs. Excess caffeine can weaken the heart muscle, while Peppermint tea has the opposite effect of strengthening the heart muscle. Coffee can hinder digestion and constipate a person, while Peppermint cleanses the entire body. Peppermint is also useful for headaches. When you have a difficult cough and mucus on the cords, add two heaping teaspoonfuls of fresh Peppermint herb to three cups of boiling water. Boil for three minutes, take off heat and let sit covered for 10 minutes. Strain and drink.

> **Note:** Research has shown that Peppermint may interfere with Iron absorption. Most herbalist agree that it should not be used by nursing mothers. In addition it is suggested to not ingest pure menthol or pure Peppermint leaves. Be careful when putting these oils into the water for inhalation, as they can burn the skin if applied in high doses.

Pleurisy Root

Pleurisy Root is excellent for all chest disorders. Its most prevalent use is for treating pleurisy, a condition that causes inflammation of the membranes surrounding the lungs. It is one of the best herbs for breaking up colds and releasing mucus. It works by reducing inflammation of the pleural membranes of the lungs and enhances secretion of healthy lung fluids. Pleurisy Root is best for those suffering from asthma and for voice professionals who have difficulty with deep breathing and inadequate air supply to the lungs when singing or speaking. Pleurisy is considered by some herbalists to be the best herb to use for colds with postnasal drip and chest congestion with mucus buildup. To make a tea, add two tablespoons to one pint of boiling water. Let brew covered for three to five minutes, and then let sit covered on low heat for 15 minutes. Strain well and drink. Drink three cups per day for one week. Add honey or Stevie to sweeten the taste.

Propolis

Propolis is a resinous mixture that honey bees collect from tree buds, sap flows, or other botanical sources to coat their hives. This amazing natural medicine has been touted as having equal or more antibacterial properties than penicillin as well as antiviral and anti-inflammatory effects. In fact, research done by Russian scientists has led them to call Propolis the "Russian Penicillin." Unlike antibiotics, it will not destroy the friendly bacteria in your gut. It is excellent for reducing swelling in the throat, breaking up mucus in the sinuses, relieving hoarseness, and fighting infection in the throat. It is safe enough to take daily to enhance the immune system and boost overall energy. Take two capsules twice a day or eat a full teaspoon of raw Propolis to stay healthy and vibrant. If you are experiencing difficult throat issues, put a large tablespoon of raw Propolis mixed in a tea of equal parts Sage, Rosemary and Myrrh (a dropper of each is a good amount). Make sure the water is not boiling hot; only use warm water for raw Propolis. Gargle three times with the liquid, swallowing after you gargle. Then drink the tea.

Rhodiola
Rhodiola is also known to herbalists as Golden Root. Its use in traditional herbal healing is noted as far back as 2000 years. Praise of this herb is worldwide from the Native Americans to China and Russia. The main use for Rhodiola is to increase physical endurance, mental performance, memory, attention span, stamina, and strength. Russia has been the only country to do extensive studies with Rhodiola. Tests done on students during exam times showed significant improvement on test scores due to an easier ability to recall information after taking Rhodiola. In addition, athletes in swimming, track, and speed skating showed rapid improvement in speed and strength. Many people have also praised Rhodiola for its ability to combat depression, using it regularly instead of prescription antidepressants. Rhodiola helps to boost the immune system by improving blood circulation and enhancing the cardiovascular system, allowing for easier and fuller breathing. This herb is outstanding for singers. I use it on a regular basis. One capsule twice a day is perfect for increasing overall energy. It can be taken one hour before performance time for an energy boost.

Rock Rose
Rock Rose has been a favorite of traditional herbalists for treating scrofula (swelling of the lymph glands), especially around the neck. This may be due to its amazing strength as an antioxidant. It also has the ability to detoxify the body of chemicals and pollutants due to smoking and pollution. Rock Rose is excellent for the immune system, as it improves and supports healthy bacterial flora. It has a very strong effect on influenza and contains antiviral properties. Given its strength, you may see why Rock Rose is very good at soothing a sore throat. Another great use for this tea is as an exterior wrap or healing compress for a sore and tired throat. For a wrap, make a strong tea

with two tablespoons of Rock Rose, one tablespoon of Echinacea, and 1/2 tablespoon of Goldenseal in one pint of boiling water for three to five minutes. Take off heat and let sit covered for 15 minutes. Take a small, clean cotton towel large enough to wrap around your neck and let it soak in the tea for 20 minutes. After soaking, slightly wring out the towel, but not so much that you lose the concentration of the formula in the towel. Wrap the warm (not too hot) towel around your neck for 10 minutes or until it becomes cool. You can keep your neck warm and the heat in the towel longer as well as avoid excess drip from the liquid by wearing a scarf around the wrap. Soak the towel again for five minutes in the tea and use as a wrap for an additional 10 minutes.

Sage

Sage is often referred to as a "cure all." It stimulates the nervous system and digestive tract. To heal ulcers in the throat, combine Sage with Myrrh, Lemon and Honey. Gargle three times a day. This is also a good remedy for aiding the healing and recovery of tonsillitis. It is effective for all throat maladies when combined with Red Root and Wood Betony. When using Sage as a tea, it should not be boiled. Steep on warm heat and keep covered while steeping. Steep two tablespoons in one pint of hot water for five minutes. Strain and drink two to three times for up to one week.

> **Note:** Most herbalists advise not to take Sage if you are a nursing mother, an individual with seizure disorders, or are pregnant.

Saw Palmetto

Saw Palmetto is most commonly used for treating urinary tract problems and BPH (benign prostatic hypertrophy), which is an age-related enlargement of the prostate gland. It has also been used over the centuries for its ability to stimulate the body's healing process when recuperating and moving into recovery after sickness, giving the body vitality and strength. In addition, it is a valuable herb for all throat problems, especially when the throat is irritated and painful. It can be used when there is excessive mucus discharge from the sinuses, throat, and nose due to its expectorant qualities, making it a wise choice when dealing with asthma and bronchial issues. If you have a sore throat due to coughing or clearing of mucus, brew up two tablespoons of Saw Palmetto in one pint of boiling water. Boil covered for three to five minutes. Steep covered for 10 minutes. Strain and gargle warm. Add a pinch of Cayenne and one tablespoon of Honey. Gargle three times, swallowing each gargle, then drink the rest of the tea. You can do the same with a liquid extract by adding one dropper full of extract in place of two tablespoons of the herb.

Schisandra
Schisandra is commonly used in Chinese medicine. Traditionally, it was used for respiratory ailments such as coughs and asthma. Modern use of Schisandra has been focused on its adaptogenic qualities, helping the body to deal with and combat stress, anxiety, and weakness. Simultaneously, it enhances mental and physical performance, positively stimulating the entire body. This has been tested successfully with athletes, soldiers, and even airline attendants. In these cases, it has been shown to significantly improve and increase stamina and concentration as well as decrease fatigue and recovery time. A good time to use Schisandra is when you are traveling or undergoing heavy performance and/or rehearsal schedules. Mix a dropper full of extract into a cup of Rock Rose tea three times a day, an hour or so before rehearsal time and airline flights.

Note: Make sure you eat some food before taking Schisandra, as it has has been known to cause slight abdominal tension when taken on an empty stomach.

Seneca (Snakeroot)
Seneca Snakeroot is named after the North American Seneca Indians who used it for healing rattlesnake bites. It became very popular in North America as the "go to" herb for difficult respiratory ailments such as asthma, whooping cough, bronchitis, pleurisy, and pneumonia. The Indian tribes used to make Seneca into an expectorant tea for sore throats due to infection. It soon became a common ingredient in cough syrups, lozenges, and cold remedies. It

has a stimulant action on the bronchial mucous membranes, promoting coughing up of mucus from the chest, easing difficult coughs and potential wheezing. If you are experiencing these symptoms and have mucus in the chest, Seneca can be an excellent remedy. It is best used In tea form. Bring one pint of hot water to a boil. Add two tablespoons of fresh root and boil covered for three to five minutes. Remove from heat and let sit covered for 15 minutes. Strain and drink. Repeat three times per day for a couple of days, keeping a good eye on the mucus discharge. If you begin to experience less mucus and ease of breathing, discontinue the tea.

Skullcap

Skullcap is one of the best and most powerful nerve tonics in the herbal kingdom. It can be compared to Catnip, Valerian, and Lobelia. It will produce sleep with no side effects in the morning and is good for people who tend to become overly excited. It also alleviates headaches, muscle spasms, and irritability. Some herbalists have used Skullcap to help people with addictions to drugs, alcohol and cigarettes. It may be used safely and regularly on a long term basis. A good introductory dose would be 10 drops of extract in two ounces of water before bedtime or during the day when you have nothing to do and can relax. Experiment with the dosage before you use it for performances.

Note: Obviously, do not use while driving. Some companies have mislabeled their products as Skullcap. Be careful not to use mislabeled Skullcap products, as they have been shown to cause liver damage.

Slippery Elm

Slippery Elm could be considered the throat's best friend when mucus membranes of the throat and lungs are swollen and inflamed. It is a demulcent, which means it soothes mucus membranes by creating a smooth film to cover and soothe the irritated tissue. This is why Slippery Elm is one of the best choices to help soothe and relieve a dry, irritated throat and is one of the main ingredients in most cough syrups on the market today. It is most powerful in respiratory disorders like pneumonia, bronchitis, and pleurisy. It also provides relief for urinary tract infections. It is used widely for digestive disorders, as it relieves constipation and cleans out the colon. Due to its amazing healing properties on the digestive system, some people use it for healing and relief of Crohn's disease. For relief of any cough or chest condition, use the formula in the "Chest and Lung" section under specific herbal formulas.

> **Note:** Slippery Elm is generally thought to be safe for pregnant or nursing women, though tests have not been done to prove otherwise. Due to its high mucilage content, most herbalists do not recommend taking Slippery Elm with other medication as it may interfere with absorption of these medicines.

St John's Wort

St John's Wort has been used for centuries to relieve anxiety, nervousness, and depression. It is associated with John the Baptist because it supposedly bloomed on his birthday. It is known as one of the most effective natural antidepressants in the herbal kingdom. In the middle ages, it was used to treat ailments such as coughs, jaundice, and dysentery and was believed to have the power to drive away devils. Today, this wonderful herb is used primarily for mild depression and anxiety as well as an expectorant to clear phlegm from the chest. The added plus of using St John's Wort for mild depression and anxiety is that it does not carry the side effects of prescription medication. St John's Wort can be a great remedy for stage fright and performance anxiety.

> **Note:** Some studies have shown this herb to induce photo sensitivity to sunlight resulting in dermatitis, inflammation of the mucus membranes, and other toxic reactions. Most herbalists recommend that anyone taking a selective serotonin reuptake inhibitor (SSRI) should never take St John's Wort. It is a diuretic, so those with sensitive bladders should not take this herb. It should not be taken by pregnant or nursing women. Check with your doctor and a qualified herbalist before using this herb.

Thyme

Thyme has long been used regularly as a culinary herb by chefs worldwide. Thyme is rich in Thymol, a volatile oil that has been proven to have powerful antiseptic, antifungal, and antibacterial properties. This makes it very effective for boosting a weak immune system. It is especially helpful in removing mucus from the head and respiratory passages. Thyme is an excellent remedy for coughs and colds as well as for sore, swollen, infected throats. If you have a difficult cough that is spasmodic in nature, Thyme can provide immediate relief. For cough and chest congestion, drink a strong cup of Thyme tea. Brew two teaspoons of fresh herb in one pint of covered boiling water for three to five minutes. Let sit covered for 15 minutes, strain and drink. For extra punch, add one teaspoon of fresh Sage and Rock Rose tea. Add honey to taste. Liquid extract may be used as well, putting one full dropper in a cup of water or tea.

Turmeric

Turmeric is a favorite of Ayurvedic practitioners and also used frequently in Chinese medicine for treating liver and digestive problems. It is one of the most widely prescribed herbs for inflammation, due to its high level of anti-inflammatory properties with its most active ingredient, Curcumin. Because of these properties it is one of the main ingredients in the Superior Vocal Health Vocal Rescue Gargle. For an overused or tired voice, use Superior Vocal Health Vocal Rescue or any formula in the "Hoarseness, Laryngitis, and Overused, Tired Voice" section under specific herbal formulas.

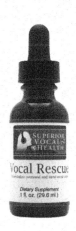

Valerian Root

Valerian or "Valeriana" comes from the Latin "valere," which means "to be in good health." Along with St. John's Root, Valerian is a commonly prescribed by herbalists because it is one of the best nerve-calming herbs. It has even been called "nature's tranquilizer." It is a safe, effective sedative for hysteria, nervous tension, stress, and insomnia. On first use, try Valerian alone in increasing doses to see how it works for you. In some people, it can have the opposite effect of acting as a stimulant. If this is the case, discontinue its use and try one of the other nerve-calming herbs such as Passion Flower or Hops. If you do choose to use Valerian, begin with 1/2 dropper of extract in a cup of warm water. You may want to add a small amount of honey for taste. Valerian tea can also be used but may not be as concentrated as the extract dose. To make your own tea, use one teaspoon of dry herb in three cups of boiling water. Boil covered for three minutes, let steep covered for 20 minutes, strain and drink. This will be a very strong cup of tea. Another plus for using Valerian as a sleep aid is that it does not interact negatively with alcohol.

Note: Most herbalists recommend not taking Valerian more than two weeks at a time. Consult with a qualified herbalist before using Valerian.

Vervain

Vervian is an herb that will produce profuse perspiration, helping to invigorate and boost the immune system. Many herbalists use it for its stimulant, astringent, and diuretic properties. It is excellent for fever reduction and is known to cure colds overnight when taken as a tea. It will expel phlegm from the throat and chest. It also strengthens the nervous system. In ancient Roman times, Vervain was chewed to heal sore teeth and gums. Vervain can be used as a restorative or recuperative remedy for the nervous system to treat nervous tension or anxiety. If you feel a chest cold coming on and phlegm developing in the chest, brew a heaping teaspoon of Vervain in a pint of covered boiling water. Boil for three minutes, then let sit covered for 15 minutes. Strain and drink about 30 minutes before going to bed. For additional support, add a dropper full of liquid extract of thyme and one dropper of Slippery Elm. Only add the extra herbs after straining.

Note: Most herbalists do not recommend taking Vervain during pregnancy because it is known to invigorate the contraction of uterine muscles during labor.

Violet

Violet is highly successful in reducing sore throats due to coughs and colds. It is also used for respiratory ailments such as bronchitis and asthma. When made into a syrup, the tea and flowers can heal mouth sores or sore gums. Violet is also used as a laxative. When combined with Nerve Root and Skullcap, it can relieve nervousness, headaches, and severe head congestion. For relief from head congestion, add two tablespoons of fresh herb to a pint of covered boiling water. Boil for three to five minutes, take off heat and let sit covered for 10 minutes. Strain and drink three cups per day for two or three days. When using a liquid extract, add 1/2 dropper of liquid extract of the herbs from the "Nerves, Anxiety, and Sleep" formula section, if you are very stressed.

Wheatgrass

Wheatgrass is an extraordinary cleanser of the entire digestive system. It is one of the best sources of immediately absorbable chlorophyll. Some studies have shown Wheatgrass to be a complete food in itself. One pound of fresh Wheatgrass has been found to be equivalent in nutritional value to 23 pounds of various vegetables. Drinking Wheatgrass helps your body build red blood cells. Every voice professional should drink an ounce or two of Wheatgrass every day for healthy, open, clean lungs and to keep the digestive tract clean and free of mucus. Wheatgrass juice protects the lungs and blood from water and air pollution, toxins, cigarette smoke, and heavy metals. It is also effective for healing a sore throat, mouth sores, and bleeding gums when used as a gargle. For these issues, rinse or gargle with 1/2 ounce of freshly squeezed Wheatgrass three times daily for one minute, then swallow. For extra healing, add a small amount of Cayenne pepper to the Wheatgrass to help absorb more quickly into your system.

White Willow

White Willow (aka White Pond Lilly) is an outstanding remedy when used for fever, headache, and inflammatory conditions such as arthritis and swollen lymph glands. It has antioxidant, antiseptic, and immune boosting effects on the body. Among its many properties,

White Willow bark contains salicin. When taken internally, salicin is slowly converted into salicylic acid, more commonly know as aspirin. Because the conversion time in the body is slow, the healing properties of White Willow continue longer than aspirin. In addition, White Willow will not upset the stomach or affect the throat negatively as aspirin can. White Willow is also useful for helping women in reducing night sweats and hot flashes. To benefit from the effects of White Willow, use 10 to 15 drops of extract in a cup of warm water up to three times a day.

Wood Sage

Wood Sage is an expectorant that is useful in the treatment of respiratory issues including tuberculosis, chest colds, and flu. It is also used to reduce inflammation of the mucous membranes of the nose and throat. If you are experiencing chest congestion, drinking Wood Sage can help loosen phlegm. Add two tablespoons of Wood Sage powdered herb to one pint of boiling water. Boil covered for three to five minutes. Take off heat and let sit covered for 15 minutes. Strain and drink. Add honey for taste. You may wish to add one tablespoon of Thyme, Seneca and Slippery Elm if you are experiencing serious congestion.

> **Note:** Most herbalists recommend not taking Wood Sage for more than three days in a row or for weeks at a time, as it has been known to increase urine and menstrual flow.

Yarrow

Yarrow is great for colds and fevers because of its anti-inflammatory, anti-allergy, and astringent properties. Hot Yarrow tea has a soothing effect on the mucus membranes, is excellent for fevers, and helps blood flow throughout the body. It increases perspiration, which helps remove toxins from the body. When combined with other respiratory and anti-inflammatory herbs such as Goldenseal, Vervain and Slippery Elm, it can break up mucus and a cold before it sets in. Add two tablespoons of Yarrow and one tablespoon of each of the previously mentioned herbs to one pint of boiling water. Boil covered for five minutes. Take off heat and let sit covered for 10 minutes.

Strain and drink while still fairly hot. Drink two cups a day. Do not drink for more than one week.

> **Note:** Most herbalists recommend not taking Yarrow during pregnancy or while nursing.

Yerba Mate

Yerba Mate is highly praised and consumed as a tea regularly throughout South America. It is quickly becoming a healthy and equally energizing substitute for coffee in the United States. Yerba Mate improves memory, stimulates digestion, fights free radicals, and stimulates the production of cortisone. It tones the entire nervous system. It is highly useful for allergies. It does contain caffeine, but only about half the amount in a cup of coffee. When purchasing this tea to brew or in tea bag form, be sure to buy it from a reputable and honest company who specializes in true Yerba Mate herb. To use as a hot tea, add one tablespoon of fresh herb to three cups of boiling water. Boil covered for three to five minutes. Take off heat and let sit covered for 10 minutes. Strain and drink warm.

> **Note:** Most herbalists suggest that Yerba Mate should not be taken by those who suffer from insomnia.

Yerba Santa

Yerba Santa is an outstanding remedy for laryngitis, bronchitis, hay fever, and asthma. It is a warming herb that has expectorant qualities. It can help remove excess mucus to help one breathe better. It is effective used as a tea when there is discharge from the nose. Because of its warming qualities, it is a good herb to take regularly during the cold and damp time of the year, especially if you will be touring or singing in cold or damp climates for extended periods of time. If on tour, keep a two-ounce bottle with you at all times. Mix a full dropper of liquid extract into a hot cup of Ginger or Sage tea, and drink once daily. If you feel a little "thick" or "cold" in the chest, drink two cups daily, one in the morning and one before going to bed.

This completes my list of the top herbs for the singer. When using any of these herbs alone or in combination, always consult an herbal practitioner first. Find out if you have any allergies to specific herbs, and always test the effect of the herb in small portions before taking a larger dose.

CHAPTER THREE
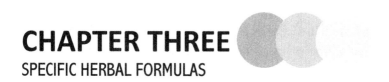
SPECIFIC HERBAL FORMULAS

The formulas listed below are for specific ailments or vocal issues. Unless otherwise noted, for efficiency, effectiveness and timing, the herbs listed in each formula are to be used as liquid extract mixed in either water or the liquid of your choice. Some herbs taste more harsh than others, so a liquid such as apple juice or something similar is recommended to curb the taste and sweeten up the mixture. You'll also notice that I have suggested various teas to be used when taking the formulas. These teas are suggested for further enhancement and healing action of the formula.

When an herb is to be brewed as a tea, follow the instructions given in the herbal section under the specific herb. You may use these herbs and formulas and adapt them as you experiment with each formula.

ALLERGY AND SINUS CONGESTION FORMULAS

1. **Cayenne, Echinacea, Garlic oil, Goldenseal, Horseradish, Boneset, Honey**

Mix a full dropper of each herb extract together in a cup or small bowl. Be sure the container is able to handle the liquid so it does not spill. Add a tablespoon of organic raw honey. If you need to heat the honey slightly to make it into a liquid, do so, but do not heat it to a boiling point or you will "kill" its healing agents. Mix all the contents well. Take a full dropper or teaspoonful of the new mixture and drop it onto the back of your tongue. Hold it for 30 seconds and let the fumes of the mixture seep up into your head. Swallow after 30 seconds. This formula may be used up to four times a day for a week. Allow for at least three hours in between each use.

2. **Brigham Tea, Burdock, Cayenne, Garlic, Goldenseal, Marshmallow, Parsley**

Brew up a strong cup of Brigham tea as instructed in the herbal section. After the tea is brewed, put in 1/2 dropper of each of the herbs. This formula is most effective when used in the morning because Brigham tea can stimulate the nervous system. Do not drink more than two cups a day and do not drink before sleeping.

3. Fenugreek, Slippery Elm, Thyme, Horseradish, Sage
Use 1/2 dropper of each herb in combination with a suggested tea. This formula is excellent for Allergies, Hay Fever, Mucus, and Sinus Congestion. Drink three cups a day for a week.
Suggested Teas: Elderberry, Blue Violet, Anise, Rock Rose

4. Goldenseal Powder
Take a small amount of Raw Goldenseal Powder about the size of half a thumbnail. Put it either on your thumbnail or on a spoon. Sniff it up into each nostril--the same amount for each side. You will feel a small stinging sensation as your sinuses get used to the powder. Let the powder sit in the nasal passages to do its work. Do not clear your nose or rinse out. The herb powder will eventually dissolve into your nasal passages, healing and clearing out potential infection or clogging. Do not do this more than one time per day, and no more than three times per week, every other day. This is a very intense and powerful procedure. Do not do this unless you are prepared for it. It is not for the weak at heart!

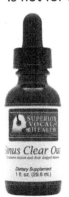

5. Sinus Clear Out
Sinus Clear Out from Superior Vocal Health is highly recommended for all sinus issues and also as a daily vocal maintenance formula. It has a highly concentrated sinus-focused formula including horseradish, cayenne, and garlic oils. You may purchase Sinus Clear Out directly from the Superior Vocal Health website, superiorvocalhealth .com.
~Also see "Eucalyptus Clear Out" in the "What do I do When" section for Sinus Congestion~

COLD AND FLU FORMULAS
1. Cayenne, Camomile, Goldenseal, Osha, Rose Hips, Sage, Yarrow

2. **Elecampane, Garlic, Parsley, Rose Hips, Rosemary, Thyme, Watercress**
3. **Garlic, Cayenne, Horseradish, Echinacea, Goldenseal, Ginger**
Use 1/2 dropper of each herb in combination with a suggested tea. Drink three cups a day for one week. These formulas are excellent for Head Colds and Flu.
Suggested Teas: Bayberry, Burdock, Rock Rose, Sage, Yarrow

4. Sinus Clear Out
Sinus Clear Out from Superior Vocal Health is highly recommended for colds and flu. It is loaded with immune enhancing herbs such as echinacea, goldenseal, olive leaf, osha and yarrow. Taken daily during a cold or flu, it will seriously help speed healing and recovery. You may purchase Sinus Clear Out directly from the Superior Vocal Health website, superiorvocalhealth.com.

ENERGY AND ENDURANCE FORMULAS
1. **Alfalfa, Bee Pollen, Cayenne, Ginseng, Gotu Cola, Licorice, Safflower**
2. **Ashwagandha, Astragalus, Gotu Cola, Ginger, Ginseng, Cayenne**
3. **American Ginseng, Cayenne, Ginger, Ginko, Propolis, Rhodiola**
All of these formulas are excellent for energy and stamina. They may be taken as a full dropper with a cup of hot water or the suggested teas and a tablespoon of honey. Drink 20 minutes before performing as well as in the middle of a show or presentation.
Suggested Teas: Astragalus, Green Tea, Gotu Cola, Peppermint, Yerba Mate,

4. Pre-show Energy Drink
Brew one tablespoon of organic green tea for five minutes on low heat. Add one dropper of Ginseng, 1/2 dropper of Gotu Cola and a teaspoon of Royal Jelly or raw Propolis. Royal Jelly is a powerful combination of Propolis extract, bee pollen, Korean Ginseng, honey and Euthero (also known as Siberian Ginseng, a lesser powerful ginseng than Korean Ginseng which helps fight stress and support adrenal gland function). This combination is excellent for the vocal cords, focus, as well as sustained and balanced energy.

HOARSENESS, LARYNGITIS AND OVERUSED, TIRED VOICE FORMULAS
1. **Goldenseal, Licorice, Marshmallow, Sage, Slippery Elm**
2. **Aloe, Cayenne, Echinacea, Garlic, Thyme, Turmeric**
3. **Ginger, Hyssop, Licorice, Myrrh, Origanum, Sage**

These formula combinations are most effective when used as a gargle. Put 1/2 dropper of the extract into two or three ounces of warm water. Make sure the water is not too hot so it does not burn your throat and cords. Mix well and gargle three times or until the mixture is finished, approximately 30 seconds each gargle. Spit out after each gargle. Adding honey to any of these formulas is also very effective and helpful. If you are experiencing difficulties with a sore throat and overused voice and must perform, gargle a few minutes before you have to sing or present as well as during your performance if possible. Gargle afterward and one more time before you go to bed so the herbs can sit on your throat overnight as you sleep. Gargle again when you wake up. Use as many times as needed.

4. Vocal Rescue from Superior Vocal Health
This formula contains almost every herb listed here in this section and is one of the most powerful and effective formulas for overused, tired voices. You may purchase Vocal Rescue directly from the Superior Vocal Health website, superiorvocalhealth.com.

5. Grandma's Old Standard
If you are unable to find the herbs above, you can always rely on the old standard, which is helpful but not as powerful in reducing inflammation or restoring the injured cords and throat. This is the combination of salt water, lemon juice, Honey and Cayenne pepper. Use one tablespoon of salt, a good squeeze of lemon, a tablespoon of honey and a pinch of cayenne pepper. Gargle the same as instructed above. This formula is good for hoarseness, laryngitis and an overused, tired voice.

CHEST AND LUNG FORMULAS

1. **Elecampane, Marshmallow, Mullein, Slippery Elm**
2. **Chickweed, Lobelia, Mullein, Osha, Sage**
3. **Elecampane, Garlic, Horehound, Nettle, Oil Of Oregano (five drops)**

Add 1/2 dropper of liquid extract of the formulas above to a suggested tea. Drink three cups per day for one week. These formulas are excellent for Lung Congestion, Bronchitis, Mucus and Phlegm in the Chest.

Suggested Teas: Seneca, Sage, Rock Rose, Pleurisy Root.

4. Dave's Lung Kicker

Here is a knockout formula for a chest cold that is very strong but palatable. Add one heaping spoonful of Pleurisy Root, Nettle, Sage and Myrrh to a pint of boiling water. Let boil covered for three to five minutes. Remove from heat and let sit covered for 20 minutes. Strain and drink. When you drink this mixture, add a pinch of Cayenne either in powder form or five drops of liquid extract. If you are feeling brave, add five drops of Horseradish extract as well. Drink this tea two times a day for three days.

5. Lung Flush

Mixing Yarrow, Plantain leaves/flowers and Coltsfoot is excellent for inhalation through steaming. In a large pot, put two pints of water and bring to a boil. Turn off heat and add 1/2 cup of each of the above mentioned herbs. Let steep on very low heat for about an hour, or 90 minutes for an extra strong dosage. Put a towel over your head and inhale the fumes deeply into your lungs. Ten minutes should be ample enough to allow the herbs to do their job. Save the brew in the pot or a glass container and store it in the refrigerator. It may be used for up to three days, three times a day for steaming.

IMMUNE BOOSTING FORMULAS

1. **Cayenne, Echinacea, Goldenseal, Honeysuckle, Oregano Oil (five drops), Propolis**
2. **Astragalus, Cayenne, Garlic, Horseradish, Onion, Red Root**
3. **Angustifolia Root, Garlic, Ginger, Goldenseal, Spilanthes**

Brew any of the teas as instructed in the herbal section. Add one dropper full of each herb extract from one of the formulas. Drink mixture three times per day for one week.

Suggested Teas: Rock Rose, Chickweed, Cinnamon, Ginger, Green Tea

4. Fasting for Immunity

Another excellent way to keep your immune system strong is "liquid fasting." This may be done with water, juice, or herbs. Doing a small one or two day fast once a month is an excellent way to keep your immune system strong and healthy. Fasting not only cleans out the toxins and mucus from your body, it also allows your digestive system to take a break and use the energy reserved for digestion to heal the areas in your body that are in need of attention, especially your immune system. There are an endless supply of books and information on the various fasts that can be done. Do your homework, and make sure the time is right to begin your fast. If done correctly and regularly, fasting can be of extraordinary benefit to keeping your immune system healthy and strong.

5. Sinus Clear Out

Sinus Clear Out from Superior Vocal Health is highly recommended for boosting and supporting the immune system. It is loaded with immune enhancing herbs such as echinacea, goldenseal, olive leaf, osha and yarrow. Taken daily during a cold or flu will seriously help speed healing and recovery. You may purchase Sinus Clear Out directly from the Superior Vocal Health website superiorvocalhealth.com.

NERVE, ANXIETY AND SLEEP FORMULAS

1. **Black Cohosh, Hops, Lemon Balm, Mistletoe, St. John's Wort, Valerian**
2. **Catnip, Hops, Lady's Slipper, St. John's Wort, Skullcap, Valerian**
3. **Evening Primrose, Hops, Kava Kava, Passion Flower, Skullcap, Valerian**

Use five to ten drops of each herb extract from one formula in a strong cup of tea. For help with sleep, drink 30 minutes before going

to bed. These formulas can be very strong and bring on sleep. If you use a full dropper, use them only for sleep. These three formulas are excellent for Headache, Stress, Nervousness and Insomnia.
Suggested Teas: Chamomile, Borage, Lavender, Hawthorn.

4. Performance Anxiety and Nervousness

The herbs in these formulas are excellent for pre-show or performance anxiety and nerves; however, do not use the full dosage amounts. Begin by using five drops of each herb in a suggested tea to monitor how you physically react. You do not want to be completely knocked out for a show or presentation. Test these formulas at lower doses before a rehearsal or at home when you are practicing on your own.

5. Stage Fright

Stage Fright from Superior Vocal Health is an excellent remedy for nerves and anxiety. It contains GABA (gamma-Aminobutyric acid) and Theanine.

Some have called GABA (gamma-Aminobutyric acid) the brain's natural anti-anxiety medicine. It is a key chemical in the brain that helps control the brain's rhythmic theta waves. Gaba may help the brain maintain physical and mental balance. Small amounts of GABA deficiency may negatively affect an individual's ability to manage even the most low-level stressful situations. This is crucial for the voice professional. Stress and anxiety are one of the main factors that can affect the quality and clear delivery of one's voice.

L-Theanine is a naturally occurring amino acid that is found in green tea. It may help to raise GABA levels. L-Theanine may also aid in promoting a calm mood in people. Additional benefits of L-Theanine are that while it may help to induce calm and ease anxiety, it also may help to promote a clearer mind, mental clarity and focus without making you tired or drowsy. When combined, GABA and L-Theanine are extremely effective at calming the brain and helping relax the entire body and nervous system. To see how these supplements affect you, start with trying 200 milligrams of L-Theanine and 100 milligrams of GABA. If this is effective and you sense yourself more at ease, take the combination before rehearsals and then gradually move it into your routine 20 minutes before a show or presentation.

You may purchase Stage Fright directly from the Superior Vocal Health website, superiorvocalhealth.com.

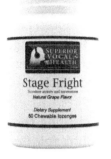

These are only a few of the many different herbal combinations that I have used. Experiment on your own and see what works for you. If you do not have the time or energy to find these herbs and mix them together, almost all of the herbs mentioned above can be found in the formulas available through superiorvocalhealth.com.

CHAPTER FOUR
SINUS HEALTH

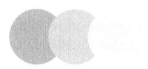

It is not enough to drink or take an herbal combination or tea. There is another important vocal health issue that needs to be addressed: Sinus health. Although we do have herbal combinations for opening and draining the sinuses, another technique that I feel promotes superior vocal health is sinus flushing. The best way to flush the sinuses is by using the Neti Pot.

Historically, Neti Pots were used in yoga to assist in clearing the nasal passages, since controlled breathing plays a central role in yoga.

The general use of a Neti Pot requires mixing a saline solution (salt and water) that will be poured through the nasal passages. You may also use a small portion of Goldenseal and Echinacea liquid extract as well. If you are really intense and adventurous, try a few drops of Cayenne in the mix. This will clean you out like nothing you have ever experienced. This combination will speed up the healing of infected nasal passages, successfully clearing them out. Use of a Neti Pot has been shown to be an effective treatment for hay fever, sinusitis and other nasal conditions. Both isotonic and hypertonic saline can be used for the Neti Pot.

GENERAL USAGE FOR THE NETI POT
1. Mix 1/4 teaspoon of finely ground, non-iodized saline solution or sea salt. Use the purest salt available as impurities in the salt can be irritating. Use lukewarm water so you don't burn your sinus passages. For Echinacea and Goldenseal mixture, use five drops of each.
2. Lean forward and turn your head to one side over the sink, keeping the forehead at the same height as the chin or slightly higher.
3. Gently insert the Neti Pot spout into the upper nostril so it forms a comfortable seal.
4. Raise the Neti Pot gradually so the saline solution flows in through your upper nostril and out through the lower nostril. Breathe through your mouth.

5. When the Neti Pot is empty, face the sink and exhale vigorously without pinching the nostrils.

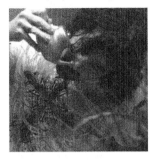

6. Refill the Neti Pot and repeat on the other side. Again, exhale vigorously to clear the nasal passages.

You should seriously start a daily regimen of sinus flushing using a Neti Pot. If you want to maintain superior vocal health, it is as important to your voice to flush your sinuses as it is to brush your teeth.

CHAPTER FIVE
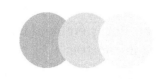

PRESCRIPTION MEDICATION, DRUGS AND THEIR EFFECTS ON THE THROAT AND VOICE

To be in superior vocal health, you must be aware of detrimental situations as well, which is why I am addressing prescription and over-the-counter (OTC) drugs. There are thousands of medications available today both through prescription and over the counter. According to the American Academy of Otolaryngology-Head and Neck Surgery, "Most medications affect the voice by drying out the protective mucosal layer covering the vocal cords. Vocal cords must be well-lubricated to operate properly; if the mucosa becomes dry, speech (and singing) will be more difficult."

In addition to the effect of chemicals and medications on the voice, their effect on the body can be just as detrimental. The liver is one of the most important organs in our body for metabolizing or breaking down medications. The more chemicals we place in our body, the more energy it takes for the liver to break down and get rid of these chemicals. Due to their toxicity, the body interprets non-natural chemicals as enemies of the system.

The body begins to immediately attack the medications, although they are supposed to be helping one symptom or another. The liver in turn has to take the valuable energy it needs to function on a normal basis and filter chemicals and debris from medications. Over time, the liver is unable to continue filtering everything, and the chemicals begin to stay in the liver, taxing it even more and robbing your body of the desired results you are naturally supposed to receive from a healthy liver. When you use herbs and a proper diet to combat colds, flu, sore throat, and other ailments affecting the voice, you are actually supporting the normal and healthy function of the liver by providing it with much needed nutrients, vitamins and minerals.

Many herbs described for the various ailments mentioned help cleanse the liver at the same time they are helping the ailments. You also will avoid the seemingly endless list of side effects that come with taking these medications. Below, you will find a partial list of some of the most frequently prescribed specific medications in the United States that research has shown to have an adverse effect on the voice and/or throat. I have listed the most commonly used drugs. They were taken directly from a more comprehensive list found at The National Center For Voice and Speech website: http://www.ncvs.org/e-learning/rx2.html.

I have also listed suggestions for natural alternatives to these medications following each medication.

Drug Group: Cardiovascular
Brand Name: Cozaar, Diovan, Hyzaar, Lotensin, Lotrol, Monopril, Prinivil, Propanolol, Vasotec, Zestoretic, Zestril, Ziac

Effect on the Voice and Throat:
Diuretics have a drying effect on mucous membranes, including those used for speaking and singing. Hoarseness, sore throat, voice changes, or laryngitis are possible symptoms. In addition to irritation effects, dry vocal cords may be more prone to injuries such as nodules.
Natural alternative: Astragalus, Brigham Tea, Chickweed, Collinsonia, Elecampane, Oil of Oregano, Osha, Propolis

Drug Group: Stimulants, brain clarity, central nervous system
Brand Name: Adderall, Ritalin
Effect on the Voice and Throat: Potential for a drying effect on vocal cord tissues which can lead to hoarseness, soreness, voice changes, or laryngitis. Additionally, dry vocal tissues may be more prone to injuries such as nodules.
Natural alternative: Ginko, Ginseng, Gotu Cola, Green Tea, Peppermint, Rhodiola.

Drug Group: Anti-asthmatic inhaled bronchodilators, anti-allergy
Brand Name: Albuterol, Atrovent, Azmacort, Combivent
Effect on the Voice and Throat: May dry or irritate tissues in the mouth and throat. May lead to hoaresness, soreness, voice changes,

or laryngitis. Dry vocal tissues may be more prone to injuries such as nodules.

Natural Alternative: Astragalus, Elecampane, Licorice root, Mullein Oil, Oregano Oil, Pau d'arco tea.

Drug Group: Antihistamines

Brand Name: Claritin, Claritin D 12 hour, Phenegran, Zyrtec, Promethazine

Effect on the Voice and Throat: Antihistamines have a drying effect on mucous membranes that may cause hoarseness, sore throat, voice changes, or laryngitis. In addition to irritation, dry vocal folds may be more prone to injuries such as nodules.

Natural Alternative: Burdock, Dandelion, Echinacea, Honey, Yerba Mate

---

Note: Get a blood test to see if you are suffering from any food allergies.

Drug Group: Sedatives

Brand Name: Ambien, Codine, Endocet, Hydrocodone, Temazepam

Effect on the Voice and Throat: The use of sedatives/narcotics may produce an uninhibited or diminished drive to speak. Symptoms of dysarthria (slow, slurred, uncoordinated speech movements) may also be linked to sedative/narcotic use.

Natural Alternative: Boneset, Catnip, Hops, Kava Kava, Lobelia, Passion Flower, Queen of the Meadow, Skull Cap, St John's Root.

Drug Group: Tricyclic antidepressants

Brand Name: Amitriptyline, Paxil, Prozac, Zoloft

Effect on the Voice and Throat: Tricyclic antidepressants may affect coordination, including the speech production system. Slow or slurred speech may be observed. They also have a drying effect on vocal fold tissues which can lead to hoarseness, soreness, voice changes, or laryngitis. Additionally, dry vocal tissues may be more prone to injuries such as nodules.

Natural alternative: Borage Oil, Calcium/Magnesium, Evening Primrose, Folic Acid, GABA, Ginko, Green Tea, Kava Kava, Lemon

Balm, Peppermint, Rhodolia, St. John's Wort, Theanine, Vitamin B-complex

Drug Group: Gastrointestinal
Brand Name: Axid, Ranitidine, Pepcid, Zantac
Effect on the Voice and Throat: The antihistamine component has a drying effect on mucous membranes which may cause hoarseness, sore throat, voice changes or laryngitis. In addition to irritation, dry vocal folds may be more prone to injuries such as nodules. However, this medication may benefit the voice if it is taken to reduce gastroesophageal reflux, as uncontrolled spillage of stomach acids into the larynx is harmful to delicate vocal fold tissues.
Natural Alternative: Drink Peppermint tea before and after meals. Aloe Vera, Acidophilus, digestive enzymes, eat more alkaline foods, proper food combining

Drug Group: Antibiotics
Brand Name: Amixcillin, Augmentin, Biaxin, Ceftin, Cefzil, Cephalexin, Cipro, Zithromax
Effect on the Voice and Throat: In general, no effects on voice or speech mechanisms are associated with antibiotic use. It should be noted, however, that antibiotic abuse can lead to an overgrowth of candida in the body, possibly leading to laryngeal thrush.
Natural Alternative: Cayenne, Colon Cleanse, Echinacea, Fresh Garlic, Goldenseal, Onion, Oregano oil, Oregamax capsules, Quercitin, Wheatgrass,

Drug Group: Steroid decongestants
Brand Name: Flonase, Flovent, Nasonex
Effect on the Voice and Throat: Throat irritation and dryness, cough, hoarseness, and voice changes are all possible effects.
Natural Alternative: Brigham Tea, Burdock, Dandelion, Echinacea, Goldenseal, Honey, Sage, Sinus Clear Out from Superior Vocal Health, Yerba Mate.

Note: Get a blood test to see if you are suffering from any food allergies.

Drug Group: Nonsteroidal anti-inflammatories
Brand Name: Ibuprofin, Naproxen, Relafen
Effect on the Voice and Throat: Vocal performers in particular should be cautious about using medications that decrease platelet function during periods of strenuous voice demands, due to an increased possibility of vocal cord hemorrhage.
Natural Alternative: Boswellin, Bromelain, Cayenne, Ginko, Ginger, Green Tea, Turmeric.

If you are a regular user of OTC medicine, you may wish to consider the alternatives listed in this chapter. If you are prescribed medication by a doctor, I am in no way suggesting or trying to convince you to quit your medicine. However, I do suggest that you seek professional advice from a health professional who is open to natural alternatives.

CHAPTER SIX
NATURAL FOOD SUPPLEMENTS

This chapter will focus on other ways to "feed" the body the nutrition that it needs to maintain superior vocal health. Natural food supplements are made up of particular foods that provide health benefits specific to that food. They may come in the form of pills, gels, granules, liquids, etc. These supplements can be quite high in certain nutrients, and in some instances may provide a combination of nutrients. The natural food supplements you will find below are listed by the area of vocal health that they affect. Some may fall under all the listed categories and some may only be under one category. No matter where they fall, all in the list are greatly needed.

The reasoning behind choosing these supplements is that I have found through my own experience and research that rarely do we have the time to eat healthy. The supplements listed are crucial for the voice professional. They have been chosen for the most pressing issues voice professionals deal with such as allergies, brain function, memory and alertness, bronchial and respiratory system, energy and fatigue, immune system building, nerves and the nervous system. These food supplements have given me a way to deal with my vocal issues and maintain a strong healthy voice, fight infections and stay vocally clear when I need to. They also provide me with plenty of extra natural energy and mental clarity. Some supplements in the list may cross over into other lists and can also be found in the herbal section as well as the food section in these chapters. For all supplements, first consult your doctor or health care provider for dosage and frequency of use.

ALLERGIES
Honey: Honey can be used for a variety of purposes. Due to its high sugar content, its most well known use is for energy. It is also helpful when combating allergies because it provides the body with minerals, B-complex vitamins, as well as vitamins C, D and E.

Note: Do not give Honey to children under the age of one because of the risk of infant botulism, which can be fatal.

Methylsulfonylmethane (MSM): This is a supplement that is mostly made up of sulphur. It has been shown to help reduce allergy symptoms and lung problems, and also boost the immune system. MSM is essential for good health and is recommended as a daily supplement.

Royal Jelly: This is a special type of milky substance created by young nurse bees. It is loaded with vitamins, including all the B-complex vitamins. It has an abundance of mineral, enzymes, hormones, amino acids, vitamins A, C and D, as well as antibiotic components. It is extremely useful for bronchial asthma and strengthens the immune system. It can be mixed with honey and kept refrigerated.
Wheatgrass: See above in the herbal section.

BRAIN FUNCTION, MEMORY AND ALERTNESS
5-HTP: This is an appetite suppressant that helps reduce food cravings as you lose weight. It assists in the metabolic breakdown of fats, carbohydrates and proteins while improving mood swings. It increases energy and naturally restores proper serotonin levels, resulting in a reduction in anxiety and depression. 5-HTP is considered a safe and effective alternative to antidepressants and anti-anxiety drugs. In fact, clinical studies have shown that it is comparable to Prozac and Valium in its ability to manage depression, anxiety, panic disorder, sleep difficulties, and many other conditions thought to be caused by chemical imbalance in the brain.

Note: Do not take 5-HTP if you are already taking antidepressant medication.

Ginkgo Biloba: See above in the herbal section.

Kelp: Kelp is seaweed and might take a little getting used to. It is available in powdered, dried, or tablet form. Kelp is rich in vitamins, including most of the B vitamins. It also contains many beneficial minerals. It is often used as a substitute for table salt. If you are not getting enough minerals in your daily diet, kelp is a good supplement to take.

Lecithin: Lecithin is an outstanding nutrient that every cell in our body needs. Lecithin is excellent for improving brain function and energy. It can be taken in capsule form, as a powder mixed in a shake or as a spread over food. It is also effective in helping the vital organs and arteries by protecting them from fatty buildup.

Melatonin: Melatonin is the hormone our body produces so we can fall asleep. At night, our Melatonin levels rise. When the sun rises, our levels fall. Some research has shown that as we age, our Melatonin levels decrease. In addition, Melatonin may help prevent hypertension and heart attack, and it also stimulates the immune system. When used as a sleep aid, it should be taken at least an hour before bedtime. At normal dosage levels, you should not wake up feeling tired or groggy as with most over-the-counter and prescription sleep medications.

Phosphatidyl Serine (PS): PS is a supplement used by every cell in the body. The brain normally produces enough PS but the levels decline with age. PS has been shown to aid the brain in memory enhancement and learning. It is best when taken with food to avoid possible nausea.

Spirulina: Spirulina is a power packed food. It can have as much as 20 times the amount of protein as soy without the dangerous digestive and hormonal side effects. It has a very positive effect on the brain and protects the immune system. It is an excellent source of chlorophyll. In addition, it can help to stimulate the appetite and at the same time cleanse and heal the entire body. It is used by most vegetarians as a source for protein while helping to stabilize blood sugar levels.

BRONCHIAL AND RESPIRATORY
Ginkgo Biloba: See above in the herbal section.

Ginseng: See above in the herbal section.

Perilla: Perilla is an Asian mint plant that has been used for centuries by Asian doctors for relief of coughs and lung problems. It is also used to combat flu and colds and to restore energy balance to the whole body.

ENERGY AND FATIGUE
Adenosine Triphosphate (ATP): ATP is a compound that has been shown to increase energy and stamina, build muscle density, increase muscle strength and energy, and delay fatigue. It is produced naturally in the body and can be an excellent source of additional support for those on the road or in situations where they are asking a lot from the body and the voice.

Alfalfa: See above in the herbal section.

Barley Grass: See above in the herbal section.

Bee Pollen: Bee Pollen is composed of 10 to 15 percent protein and also contains B-complex vitamins, vitamin C, enzymes, potassium and simple sugars. It helps fight fatigue, depression and allergies because it enhances the immune system. Some people may be allergic to Bee Pollen so try a small amount first and wait a few minutes to monitor your body reaction. If you begin to feel throat irritation or itching throughout the body, do not use.

Dimethylglycine (DMG): DMG is a safe, non-toxic food substance that does not build up in the body. It has been shown to help the body maintain high energy levels and boost mental acuity under stressful situations. It has also been found to enhance the immune system. Most important, it improves oxygen utilization by the body helping to normalize blood pressure. It is effective when used 10 to 15 minutes before a performance because it gives the voice an additional boost through natural energy. DMG is one of the ingredients found in Stage Fright from Superior Vocal Health. You may purchase Stage Fright directly from the Superior Vocal Health website, superiorvocalhealth.com.

Ginseng: See above in the herbal section.

Honey: See above in the herbal section.

Inosine: Inosine is naturally produced by the body. It helps in the transportation of oxygen to muscle cells resulting in the production of energy. It is used often by weight lifters and body builders to increase muscle and support the immune system.

> **Note:** Inosine should not be taken by those who have kidney problems or gout.

Kombucha Tea: Kombucha tea is a rare form of tea made from the mushroom itself. It has detoxifying properties and is known to be a natural energy booster.

Octacosanol: This is an oil concentrate made of naturally derived wheat germ. It is a fabulous supplement that has been proven to increase oxygen utilization during exercise thus increasing physical endurance, reaction time and tissue oxygenation. In addition, it helps reduce blood cholesterol levels.

Perilla: See above.

Spirulina: See above in the herbal section.

Wheatgrass: See above in the herbal section.

IMMUNE SYSTEM BOOSTING
Bee Pollen: See above.

Chlorella: Chlorella contains high levels of chlorophyll, which is one of the main agents used in keeping our bodies in proper acid/alkaline balance. It contains a tremendous amount of natural protein (almost

58 percent), all of the B vitamins, vitamins C and E, and rare trace minerals. It can be considered almost a complete food. Studies have shown that chlorella is an excellent source of protein, especially for vegetarians.

Corn Germ: Corn Germ is made from isolating the embryo of the corn plant. It is high in zinc, containing 10 times the amount found in wheat germ.

Dimethylglycine (DMG): See above.

Garlic: See above in the herbal section.

Inosine: See above.

Kombucha Tea: See above.

Lecithin: See above.

Methylsulfonylmethane (MSM): See above.

Royal Jelly: See above.

Spirulina: See above.

Wheatgrass: See above.

NERVES AND THE NERVOUS SYSTEM
Aloe Vera: See above in the herbal section.

Inosine: See above.

Melatonin: See above.

As you can see, there are many supplements which can be taken on a regular basis as needed to maintain superior vocal health. One thing to remember, however, is that no amount of supplements can replace healthy, conscientious eating. You need to be sure to eat the proper foods, and not eat improper foods that will cause you to get sick or adversly affect your vocal health.

CHAPTER SEVEN
ON-THE-RUN FOODS FOR
THE VOICE PROFESSIONAL

In this section you will find a list of foods that will enhance, invigorate, strengthen, and boost your overall energy level. These foods help support a healthy immune system, give you more mental clarity, aid in the digestive process, and keep your body clean. The goal of this chapter is to bring to your attention the myriad of alternatives available in choosing the best foods for optimal vocal health. In addition, by eating these foods more often you should see a marked improvement in your overall health.

These foods will allow you to access your true potential as a voice professional by giving your body and your voice the support it needs. Proper nutrition is one of the most important aspects of having and maintaining a healthy, full, clear and strong voice. If your body cannot supply you with the energy you need to produce the sounds you are capable of producing, you will almost always fall short vocally. I have always maintained the belief that, "You sing/speak what you eat."

If you are eating foods that create mucus, slow down and impede your digestion, cause fatigue, create indigestion and acid reflux, then you are doing all of that to your voice as well. As a voice professional, you cannot afford to do this to yourself. The food you eat is the fuel with which you deliver your voice to the world.

I have found the issue of not eating or eating improperly on the run to be one of the most pressing issues when it comes to voice professionals trying to do their craft while living unbelievably busy lives. Why compromise yourself when you don't have to? There are foods that are easy to eat, taste great and don't leave you feeling bloated or tired; and the energy they provide is even and smooth. They do not give you too much energy at one time or overload your nervous system the way caffeine, white processed sugar, white flour and carbohydrates do. Most of these foods are grown organically or produced under a more stringent quality control system, which means they are not filled with chemicals and additives.

Clearly, we need to get plenty of rest, drink lots of fresh, clean water and employ proper technique. However, when we eat foods that slow us down and fill our body and ultimately our throat, chest, and sinuses with mucus and phlegm, we run into problems that can eventually affect our health, vocal health, and career.

Most of the time, the life of the voice professional does not allow for a "regular" schedule. We are more on the run than anything else. This makes it difficult for us to get the proper nutrition we need for performing quality vocals every time we sing or present. We also do not have the time to prepare food and cook the way we might want. Fortunately, there are many stores and restaurants that can provide us with the foods you will find in this list.

When I am on the road, I go online and search the area I am traveling so I can find the stores and restaurants I need. That way I do not waste time and energy and end up eating what I don't want because I got too hungry and ate what I knew was not good for me. Make the commitment to yourself to begin eating what works for your voice and body. Eat the way you wish to sing or speak: Clear, light, colorful, strong, focused, consistent, powerful and beautiful.

Below you will find an excellent list of different "on-the-run" foods that can provide you with energy, mental clarity, strength, calmness, and overall better health. In addition, most or all of these foods will help boost your immune system, enrich your cells, and benefit your digestive system. As voice professionals, we must continually be conscious and vigilant of what we put into our body each and every time we eat. As I mentioned before, we cannot afford to call in sick. It is our responsibility to take care of ourselves and stay in an optimal health zone. Our voice is a direct reflection of our physical and mental state.

This list is the result of the last 20 years of my life researching and discovering how to give my body what it needs so it can produce the best sound. Do your own research, as well. Find out what works and what doesn't work for you. Give yourself the gift and blessing of a voice that can thrive and shine at its best, ultimately resulting in superior vocal health.

Aloe Vera Juice: This comes from the aloe plant. Aloe has been known for centuries to be an amazing healing plant and an immune system booster. Drinking two ounces of pure aloe juice daily can do wonders for your health. Aloe has been used to help enhance the body's immune system in cancer patients, while they undergo chemotherapy by promoting the growth of new and healthy cells. Drinking aloe regularly can greatly reduce acid reflux and help the digestive system to work properly and more efficient. Aloe Vera juice is easy to travel with and tastes almost exactly like regular water.

Avocado: Avocados are considered a "super fruit," containing nearly 20 vitamins, minerals, and beneficial plant compounds. They are also a great source of fiber and protein. When eaten raw, they digest well and can fill you up without making you feel overly full. Avocados are high in folate and have a good amount of potassium, both necessary for a balanced nervous system and energy.

Banana: Bananas are one of my favorite foods. I almost never travel or perform without having them in my bag. Bananas are loaded with potassium and magnesium. Both minerals provide the body with clear, focused energy. Bananas do not fill you up or create mucus in the throat or body. They are easy to travel with, very tasty, and excellent to eat before an audition, presentation or performance if you did not have time for a full meal. When I was younger and training in martial arts, if I was unable to eat before my workout my instructor would tell me to eat two bananas to carry me through the entire workout.

Beans: Beans are an excellent source of non-meat protein, folic acid which helps brain function, and soluble fiber which helps keep blood sugar under control. This is important if you are prone to emotional and physical swings due to your blood sugar levels going up and down. You do not want this happening while you are singing or presenting.

Blueberries: Blueberries are also considered a "super fruit." Studies have shown that the antioxidant properties of blueberries are the highest of all fruits. Antioxidants are substances that may protect your cells against the effects of free radicals (molecules produced when your body breaks down food), or environmental exposures like tobacco smoke and radiation, many of which can be found when on the road traveling. Free radicals can damage cells and may play a role in heart disease, cancer, and other diseases. Antioxidants also play a huge role in brain clarity, helping to keep your brain at its clearest and most focused. In addition, eating blueberries can keep you healthy and clean digestively.

Black Tea: Black tea with your breakfast, lunch or dinner is a great addition to a meal (unless you are sensitive to small amounts of caffeine). It is full of antioxidant properties, has about half the amount of caffeine, and has been shown to expand the arteries in a subtle way, thereby increasing the blood flow to the heart. Black tea is also believed to delay the aging process. It is great to drink 20 minutes before performing or presenting because the caffeine level is so low that it does not overload your brain, make you nervous, or cause you to tense or tighten up in the chest and throat. It does provide you with a quick boost of manageable energy. In addition, it will warm your body in colder climates. I drink black tea on a regular basis two or three times a day and always carry it with me when on the road.

Cacao: Most of us know cacao as chocolate. However, the chocolate from a Hershey or Snickers bar is not good for us as voice professionals because of the mix of milk, sugar, and chemical additives, making it an open invitation for mucus and digestive difficulties. Raw cacao is an excellent form of energy because it contains theobromine. Theobromine acts a lot like caffeine but without the same side effects. Studies have also found that it can reduce the rate of heart disease and improve circulation, as well as improve memory and learning. It can be eaten in the form of a bar as "nibs," or as a cacao bean.

Chia Seeds: You may know "chia" as the "Chia Pet" from television. In fact, these seeds are the same ones used for that product. However, when eaten as seeds or sprouts, they are fantastic for the body and overall health. I sprinkle them on a salad or mix them in with my spirulina and Emergen-C drink. Chia seeds actually hydrate the body from the "chia gel" thus giving us more energy. They are also the richest plant source of Omega-3 on the planet. Omega-3 is the vital fat that protects against pain and inflammation in the body and helps us move easier, allowing our energy to be more smooth and free. In addition, Omega-3 helps the brain by alleviating symptoms of depression and bipolar disease, allowing our mental energy to flow resulting in a lighter and more flowing voice.

Dried Fruit: In general, dried fruit is great for your overall health. I always keep a supply in my bag whenever I am in rehearsals. I particularly like dried mango. Mango is extremely high in potassium providing consistent energy, and it does not cause or create any mucus. I also eat dried mango 20 minutes or so before a performance or audition if I am hungry and did not get to eat a meal but don't want to fill my stomach up before I sing. Some other energizing dried fruits are raisins, apples and bananas.

Emergen-C: Emergen-C is a product that I use daily even when I am not singing, performing, or auditioning. It is a great source of quick energy when you need it. It is an excellent source of vitamin C with 1000 mg per serving. It also has a decent amount of potassium, vitamin B, zinc, and magnesium (all supplements we need for maintaining energy), and it is good for the immune system. Emergen-C packets are easy to carry around, easy to use, and taste great. They come in various flavors and you only need a bottle or cup of water to mix with it. I start each day with two packets as part of my breakfast, and I'm never without them when I'm on the road or performing.

Energy Bars: Energy bars come in all shapes and sizes, and there is an endless supply of excellent ones from which to choose. A live, organic energy bar can provide more nutrients, minerals, vitamins, and protein than a meal from McDonalds or Subway and certainly more than a Snickers bar. Make sure you get a bar that is live and organic. I always keep these with me when I'm on the road; that way I know I'm getting all the nutrition I need in case I don't have time to eat. They also taste great, do not cause mucus to build up in the throat or sinuses, and are very good for healthy digestion. Make sure you find bars that are not loaded with caffeine or sugar.

Figs: Figs have been eaten as a delicacy since Roman times, probably due to the fact that they contain two nutritional properties that make you feel good: Potassium and tryptophan. Eating only six figs can provide up to 891 mg of potassium, an amount comparable to that found in a large banana. They are also very rich in fiber. Tryptophan helps the body relax and is often used by people with sleep disorders. Figs also contain large amounts of calcium, also a relaxing agent.

Fruit: As a general reminder, almost all fresh fruit is excellent for providing quick energy. If you are prone to sugar swings, eat some sort of good fat with your fruit, such as avocado or nuts. This will help to buffer the speed at which the sugar enters your blood stream. Bananas and mango are high in potassium and are needed for energy. Pineapple is good for the throat if you are having swelling or soreness, as it contains bromelain which helps to reduce inflammation.

Orange Energy Drink: If you have time to prepare something at home and bring it with you, try this fruity super energy drink. It is a favorite and original from David Wolfe, one of the foremost experts on raw food dieting. Take two oranges and 1/2 cup of ice and blend them. This alone is a tremendous energy booster. I have added one tablespoon of flax seed oil and a tablespoon of almond butter. Keep it in an insulated bottle and drink it about 20 minutes or so before your presentation or audition. The oranges will provide you with an enormous amount of energy, while the almond butter will buffer the sugar going into your blood and the flax seed oil will balance out the chemicals in your brain, thereby allowing you to relax and focus.

Ginger: Ginger when eaten raw is an amazing food for the voice. For starters, when sucked on like a piece of candy it promotes salivation and can keep you from getting a dry throat and mouth. If you chew on it slowly, it is excellent for warming up the throat, vocal cords and chest. Heat in these areas will help to invigorate without overloading and causing trauma to your vocal mechanism. Ginger is also outstanding for heating the entire body if you are traveling, singing, or presenting in colder climates. Eat it every day to keep the energy in your entire body warm and fired up. It is also excellent for digestion and helps keep the whole digestive tract clean and free of unwanted debris.

Gogi Berries: Gogi Berries are a tasty and energizing snack when you need quick energy. They are loaded with vitamin C and potassium. As a dried fruit they are easy to keep in your bag and do not require refrigeration.

Green Tea: See above.

Himalayan Goji Juice: Himalayan Goji Juice has been used for all kinds of healing of the body and for almost any ailment. It is one of the most amazing sources of vitamins and minerals you can get in one food. A cup of Himalayan Goji juice contains more protein than whole wheat, as well as B-complex, vitamins, up to 21 minerals needed for energy and focus, and 500 times the amount of vitamin C by weight than oranges. It tastes great and can easily be transported in a bag or briefcase. I highly recommend it for daily use and on the road.

Nuts (sprouted): Nuts are an excellent source of protein that will not make you feel stuffed or full like a hamburger or a slice of pizza. They are excellent to eat when you have not been able to get a meal before an audition or presentation. Make sure you get nuts that are raw. Try not to eat roasted or salted nuts as they are often difficult to digest. My favorites have been almonds, sunflower seeds and pumpkin seeds. If you want an extra benefit from nuts, try sprouting them. As I mentioned before, un-sprouted nuts are difficult to digest. Sprouting nuts makes them a live food, enabling the enzymes and nutrients to be more readily available and easier to digest. When sprouted, nuts increase in protein and decrease in carbohydrates. An added benefit is that they also taste great sprouted. Sprouting nuts is easy. Pour a cup of raw nuts into a bowl and fill it with good filtered water. Let it sit for eight hours or overnight. Drain the water and dry them off. Put them in the refrigerator because they are now "live." If you are going to keep them in your bag or lunch, use an insulated bag and ice pack for traveling.

Raisins: Raisins are tasty, easy to travel with, and provide energy. They are good for your brain because they are an excellent source of boron, a trace element that improves hand/eye coordination, attention, and memory. Raisins do not fill you up and can be combined with various nuts for a well balanced, high energy snack. My favorite combination has always been raisins and sprouted almonds.

Seaweed: Seaweed is a food that does not overfill you, slow you down, create mucus, or make you tired. It is easy to travel with, and you can keep it in your bag for quick consumption. In addition, it is loaded with vitamins and minerals, especially B vitamins which help you deal with stress and can provide energy and mental clarity. Seaweed has been shown to enrich the bloodstream, assist the metabolism, and warm the body. This is especially important if you are singing or presenting in colder climates.

CHAPTER EIGHT
PROPER ACID/ALKALINE BALANCE

One of the most important factors that determines our vocal health is maintaining a balanced acid/alkaline level in the body. If we can maintain this balance most of the time, we can pretty much depend on our voice and body staying healthy, thereby avoiding sickness such as colds, flu, mucus in the throat, chest and lungs, and other throat and respiratory afflictions. An acidic body contributes to suppressed immune functions, and this could be considered the number one reason for overproduction of mucus in the body.

The balance between acid and alkaline is described by the term pH or "potential of hydrogen concentration." The ideal pH is 7.0 to 7.2. When our pH balance is at optimal levels, it is almost impossible for disease to exist in the body; the reason for this is that when the body is in an ideal pH state, it is full of oxygen, the cells are being energized, and the immune system is strong and able to fight off most infection.

On the other hand, when the body is overly acidic, all kinds of diseases can show up. An overly acidic body can be responsible for simple issues such as fatigue, tension, depression, acid reflux, sinus problems or allergies. On an even more serious side, an overly acidic body can lead to poor circulation, gout, ADD, seizure disorders and even cancer. You may check your pH level easily in the comfort of your own home with litmus paper strips. These can be purchased at any health food store or online. The test is easy and quick. Simply follow the directions on the package.

Poor dietary choices are the number one reason the body becomes overly acidic. One of the main reasons that most people are in this state is due to a diet high in meats, caffeine, sugar, processed foods, white flour, glutens, and carbonated beverages. In fact, the acid level in carbonated beverages is extremely high—so high that it can take up to 30 cups of water to neutralize the acid level from one can of soda. In addition to eating the proper foods, another way to neutralize some of the acid in your body is to drink plenty of good filtered water on a regular basis.

Below you will find two lists: Foods that can lead to an alkaline state in the body--"General Alkaline Producing Foods"--and foods that can lead to an acidic state in the body--"Acidifying Foods." These lists contain general foods, spices, seasonings, minerals, and "other" sources that are categorized as alkaline or acid. The determination for this list is based on the type of residue that remains after the food is digested. In addition, there is a list that contains some foods which can be attributed to either being alkaline or acid. Ultimately we want to eat a minimum of 80% alkaline foods on a daily basis.

General Alkaline Producing Foods
Alfalfa, Almonds, Apples, Apricots, Avocado, Bananas, Barley Grass, Beans, Beets, Green Beets, Berries, Blackberries, Broccoli, Brussels Sprouts, Cabbage, Cantaloupe, Carrots, Cauliflower, Celery, Chard Greens, Cherries (sour), Chestnuts, Chlorella, Coconut, Fresh, Collard greens, Cucumbers, Currants, Dandelions, Dates (dried), Dulce, Figs (dried), Eggplant, Garlic, Grapefruit, Grapes, Green Beans, Green Peas, Honeydew Melon, Kale, Kohlrabi, Lettuce, Lemon, Limes, Millet, Molasses, Mushrooms, Musk Melons, Mustard Greens, Nectarine, Onions, Oranges, Parsnips, Peaches, Pears, Peas, Peppers, Pineapple, Pumpkin, Radishes, Raisons, Raspberries, Rhubarb, Rutabagas, Sauerkraut, Sea Vegetables, (Nori, Wakame), Spinach (green), Spirulina, Sprouts, Strawberries, Sweet Potatoes, Tangerines, Tempeh (fermented), Tofu (fermented), Tomatoes, Watercress, Watermelon, Wheatgrass, Whey Protein Powder, Wild Greens.

Alkaline Spices and Seasonings
Chili Pepper, Cinnamon, Curry, Ginger, Herbs (all), Miso, Mustard, Sea Salt, Tamari.

Alkaline Minerals
Calcium, Cesium, Magnesium, Potassium, Sodium.

"Other" Alkalizing foods
Alkaline antioxidant water, Organic Apple Cider Vinegar, Bee Pollen, Fresh Fruit Juice, Green Juices, Lecithin, Blackstrap Molasses, Probiotic cultures, Soured Dairy Products, Vegetable Juices.

Acidifying Foods

Alcoholic beverages, Almond Milk, Amaranth, Bacon, Barley, Beef, Beer, Black Beans, Blueberries, Bran (oat), Bran (wheat), Bread, Butter, Canned or Glazed Fruits, Canola Oil, Carob, Carp, Cashews, Catsup, Cheese (regular and processed), Chick Peas, Clams, Cocoa, Cod, Coffee, Corn, Corn Oil, Corned Beef, Corn Syrup, Cornstarch, Crackers (soda), Cranberries, Currants, Fish, Flax Oil, Flour (wheat), Flour (white), Fried Foods (all), Green Peas, Haddock, Hard Liquor, Hemp Seed Flour, Hemp Seed Oil, Ice Cream, Ice Milk, Kamut, Kidney Beans, Lamb, Lard, Legumes, Lentils, Lobster, Macaroni, Mussels, Mustard, Noodles, Oatmeal, Oats (rolled), Olives, Olive Oil, Organ Meats, Oyster, Peanut Butter, Peanuts, Pecans, Pike, Pinto Beans, Plums, Pork, Prunes, Quinoa, Rabbit, Red Beans, Rice (all), Rice Cakes, Rice Milk, Rye, Safflower Oil, Salmon, Sardines, Sausage, Scallops, Sesame Oil, Shellfish, Shrimp, Spaghetti, Spelt, Soy Beans, Soy Milk, Sugar, Sunflower Oil, Tahini, Tuna, Turkey, Walnuts, Wheat Germ, Wheat, White Beans, Winter Squash, Veal, Venison.

"Other" Acidifying foods

Black or Red Pepper, Soft Drinks, Vinegar

Acidifying chemicals and drugs

Aspirin, Drugs (medicinal) Drugs (psychedelic), Herbicides, Pesticides, Tobacco.

For additional help with diet and how specific foods affect your body and voice, you may find outstanding information from the web sites below:

Weston A. Price Foundation, **www.westonaprice.org**

Acid Reflux: Achieving Lasting Healing with Traditional Foods, Performance without Pain—
www.performancewithoutpain.com

CHAPTER NINE
WHAT DO I DO WHEN?

I like to call this the "go to" chapter for times when you are in need of a quick remedy. It is a list of the classic scenarios I personally have faced, as have many singers, actors, teachers and speakers I have worked with. I found these remedies and formulas through research and choose the ones I felt were the most effective and applicable to help the voice professional in need.

What do I do when I wake up with clogged sinuses and have to sing that day/night?

Eye Bright Clean Up
Put two heaping spoonfuls of fresh or dried Eye Bright in one pint of boiling water. Remove from heat and let sit covered for 10 minutes. Drink several cups for nasal congestion and sinusitis. This tea has been found useful for hay fever as well as allergies to dust and pets.

Sinus Clear Out
Sinus Clear Out from Superior Vocal Health is also an outstanding formula to completely clear out and open up the sinus passages. You may purchase Sinus Clear Out directly from the website, superiorvocalhealth.com.

Sinus Opener
Take a quarter tablespoon of sea salt. Mix it with two or three pinches of Goldenseal powder and enough filtered water to form a liquid paste. Sniff the paste up into your nostrils or coat them with the mixture. Allow it to stay there as long as you are able. You may feel relief immediately if not very soon. This is due to the Goldenseal reaching the mucus membranes and its effect on the entire throat and sinus cavity.

Eucalyptus Clear Out

This is what you will need before you begin:

1) 1 bottle of quality Eucalyptus Oil.

2) 2 Q-tips

3) A warm shower

Turn on your shower to a heat you can handle without it being too hot on your skin. Put a number of towels at the bottom of the door so the steam from the shower does not escape under the door. Just steaming alone is excellent and essential for proper vocal care and when your vocal apparatus is under siege; however, this procedure will speed healing even more.

Before you get into the shower, take each Q-tip and dip it in the Eucalyptus Oil making sure it is completely covered and soaked. Put the Eucalyptus Oil and Q-tips on a clean towel or tissue on the counter next to the shower or somewhere close so you can reach them from the shower. Before you get into the shower, spill a few drops of Eucalyptus Oil on the floor of the shower. Be careful how much you use; too much oil may burn your feet, so only use a few drops.

Get into the shower and breathe deeply, slowly allowing the mixture to fill your lungs. Take a few minutes to let the steam and Eucalyptus Oil begin opening your sinus passages.

After you have allowed the steam to open you up, take one oil-soaked Q-tip and insert it into one nostril. Very gently and slowly, slide the Q-tip up into your sinus passage making sure it goes all the way up into your sinus passage as far as it can go. Next, slowly and even more gently twist and turn the Q-tip so it coats your entire sinus passage.

Now slowly pull the Q-tip out as you feel the openness in your sinus cavity and the energy of the oil working.

Take the other oil soaked Q-tip and do the same thing to your other nostril and sinus passage.

Within 30 seconds (or sooner) you will probably begin to sneeze longer and stronger than you ever have before! This is the clearing power of the oil and your sinus passages expelling all the mucus and bacteria that has been clogging you up. In addition, the oil will slide down into the back of your throat opening, cleaning, and clearing out any mucus or bacteria.

Clogged Sinuses and Peppermint

When you find yourself stuffed up and congested, use pure peppermint oil for instant relief. If you have an inhaler, mix five drops of peppermint, three drops of eucalyptus, two drops of oregano oil and two drops of tea tree oil. Inhale this mixture for five minutes. If you do not have an inhaler, boil two cups of water in a small pot. Take the water off the heat. Put the mixture of oils into the water. Cover your head with a towel and inhale the fumes for five minutes. Peppermint oil is also very good in combating viruses and bacteria. This will put you on the path to quick recovery.

What do I do when I have a constant runny nose/excess mucus and need to perform?

Runny Nose and Head Cold

In Germany, a popular remedy for runny nose and head colds in children and adults has been a tea made from walnut leaves. This tea helps dry up sinus discharge. Take two tablespoons of walnut leaves and add to one pint of boiling water. Boil for three minutes, stir and cover. Remove from heat and allow to steep for 30 minutes. One cup of the tea, lukewarm, every three hours is suitable for adults with a head cold. For children, 1/2 cup every 4 hours is suitable to help stop a runny nose.

Mucus Thinners

To thin mucus secretions, drink water every couple of hours. A good organic chicken soup with garlic or ginger and plenty of green vegetables added will bolster the immune system and thin mucus secretions. Eating onions will help, due to their anti-inflammatory properties. In addition, barley soup will reduce phlegm.

Break Up Sinusitis

Add lots of cayenne, garlic, onions, and horseradish to your meals. These will ease the pressure and aid mucus drainage. If you can handle it, eat a small spoonful or two of crushed horseradish mixed with lemon juice.

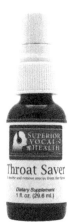

Throat Saver Spray

Throat Saver from Superior Vocal Health is designed to help remove excess mucus from the throat and open up the sinus passages with organic peppermint oil. This spray can be used all day long and can be purchased directly from the website, superiorvocalhealth.com.

What do I do if I have a sore throat and still need to perform?

Olive Oil Treatment

The ancient philosopher Homer called Olive Oil "Liquid Gold." For a sore throat or mild cough, take a small sip of Olive Oil and let it rest in your throat for a minute or two, then swallow.

Suck on Garlic

This Amish remedy can treat or prevent sore throats. Peel a fresh clove of garlic, slice it in half and place one piece in each cheek. Suck on the garlic like a cough drop. Occasionally, crush your teeth against the garlic, not to bite it in half but to release its allicin, a chemical that can kill the bacteria which causes strep throat.

Infection Fighter

Combine equal parts of Chickweed, Black Cohosh, Goldenseal, Lobelia, Skullcap, Brigham Tea, and Licorice. This helps fight infection in the body and is good when taken internally to help heal and soothe a sore throat.

Sore Throat Pain Remover

To cure a sore throat due to cold or flu, mix pinches of organic sea salt and cayenne pepper with the juice of half a lemon or lime and gargle. There may be a brief period of burning in the throat, but the soreness will quickly be gone.

Tumeric Throat Healer

Gargle with turmeric. Turmeric is one of nature's most powerful healers. The active ingredient in turmeric is curcumin. Tumeric has been used for over 2500 years in India. It is a natural antiseptic and antibacterial agent. Try this gargle to calm a cranky throat: Mix together three ounces of hot water, 1/2 teaspoon turmeric and 1/2 teaspoon salt. Gargle with the mixture twice a day. If you're not good with a gargle, mix 1/2 teaspoon turmeric in one cup hot milk and drink. Turmeric stains clothing, so be careful when mixing and gargling.

Vocal Rescue Gargle

Vocal Rescue from Superior Vocal Health is one of the most powerful and effective formulas created to help ease sore throat pain due to inflamation from over-singing, infection or sickness.

Put two full droppers in two ounces of warm water and gargle. Vocal Rescue can be purchased directly from the website, superiorvocalhealth.com.

Cayenne Clear Out

This formula is outstanding for coughs and clearing mucus. Cut one ounce or so of Slippery Elm into small pieces about the size of a small child's fingernail. Add a pinch of cayenne and some lemon for taste. Sweeten with honey and infuse into a pint of boiling water. Drink warm, 1/2 a cup or so, over a number of hours. The addition of the Slippery Elm will force the mucus to pass down through the intestines. This is also very nourishing and has excellent healing qualities for the body in general.

Rasberry Rescue

Raspberry leaf tea can make a great gargle for a sore and tired throat. Using a medium to large size mug, pour one cup boiling water over two teaspoons dried leaves. Steep for ten minutes, then strain. Allow to cool. Do not drink any liquid you have used as a gargle.

Russian Throat Cure
Combine one tablespoon of pure horseradish or horseradish root with one teaspoon honey and one teaspoon ground cloves. Mix in a glass of warm water and drink slowly.

Black Alder Miracle
Black Alder was used to dye wool in Great Britain and probably got its name from the color of its bark, although the color is more of a reddish-yellow. Apparently villagers in the countryside used to gargle with a good shot of Black Alder Bark, and it would clear up their throats as if it was a miracle!

Apple Cider Savior
This sore throat cure is found in several different remedies. Some doctors still swear that it is surprisingly palatable and works wonders. (Do not give it or any other honey-containing food or beverage to children under two years of age. Honey can carry a bacteria that can cause a kind of food poisoning called infant botulism, and it may also cause allergic reactions in very young children.) Combine one tablespoon honey with one tablespoon apple cider vinegar in eight ounces hot water. Mix all the ingredients together in a mug and sip slowly (but don't let it get cold). Use as often as desired. For gargling, you'll need one teaspoon salt, half a cup of cider vinegar, and one cup warm water. Dissolve the salt in the vinegar, then mix in the water. Gargle every 15 minutes as necessary.

The Old Salt Water Standard
If you can gargle without gagging, make a saline solution by adding half a teaspoon salt to a cup of very warm water. Yes, when your mother told you to gargle with saltwater, she knew what she was talking about. It cuts phlegm and reduces inflammation.

What do I do if I am really congested and need to perform?

Cold and Mucus Congestion Buster
One cup of Horehound tea will instantly loosen impacted

phlegm in the throat, lungs and sinuses. It also will relieve a sinus headache. To make the tea, bring one pint of hot water to a boil, then add 2-1/2 teaspoons of the fresh or dried herb and let boil for three minutes. Remove from heat, cover, and steep 45 minutes. Drink the tea while it is lukewarm with a squeeze of lemon and some honey or blackstrap molasses for taste. This tea will just about knock any cold and congestion unconscious.

Trampoline It
If you feel your glands are beginning to swell and get clogged, jump on a trampoline. The bouncing action will immediately begin to shake and clear the glands, allowing the mucus to drain out much faster. It is a good idea to jump on a trampoline daily for superior vocal health.

Chest and Throat Pleghm Relief
For relief of chest and throat phlegm, add two heaping spoonfuls of Coltsfoot herb to a pint of boiling water and boil as a tea. Moisten a cloth with the freshly made tea and apply the cloth to the chest and throat for 10 or 15 minutes. This will loosen chest and throat phlegm and is very good for coughs and bronchitis.

What do I do if I feel something coming on the night before a performance?

Flu Buster Brew
Natural Doctor Silenna Heron of Sedona, Arizona, promotes a "recovery therapy" using Boneset, equal parts of Yarrow, Elder Flower, and Lemon Balm or Peppermint combined to make a warm tea. She encourages her patients to drink a cup of this tea, get into a hot bath and then drink a second cup while still in the tub. After drying off, go straight to bed and cover up with first a sheet followed by heavy blankets and quilts. This will promote heavy sweating for one hour. Then return to the tub and sponge the body off with apple cider vinegar. According to those who have done this, "by the next morning, they were fully recovered."

Herb Burn Out

This remedy is from the Famous Dr. Schultz, "Herb Doc." I have altered it slightly but essentially it is his original remedy. I have done this before and it is extremely effective. This is excellent to do if you feel something coming on the night before or a couple of nights before a performance. Run a bath as hot as you can take it.

While the bath is running and filling up, brew up a quart of any type of herb tea. Make sure the tea does not contain caffeine. Set this container of tea next to the bathtub.

Soak a small towel in cold water. Set it next to the bathtub in arms reach as well.

Get into the bath easily, making sure you do not burn yourself. After you are in the bath, begin to drink the tea hot. As you drink, you will begin to sweat profusely. Stay in the heated bath as long as you can, making sure to drink the entire amount of tea.

Every few minutes make sure to cool yourself off with the cold towel.

At the end of the bath, drain the tub and take a shower as cold as you can stand it. Make sure to stand under the cold water for at least five minutes.

Just before you go to bed, drink a warm cup of Chamomile or Borage tea.

You should wake up the next morning feeling much better.

What do I do when I can't sleep the night before a performance or show?

Natural Tranquilizer

Calcium and magnesium work together to ease nervousness and calm your system overall, without drowsiness or causing a "foggy" head. When in an emergency or if you need to calm down quickly, powdered calcium and magnesium concentrate mixed with a glass of water is extremely effective.

Sleep Foods

If you have to eat later at night after a show or while on the road, there are specific foods that can help you sleep better. Nut butter,

Almond butter is a great choice. Tuna, turkey, whole grain crackers, and yogurt are all high in tryptophan, which promotes relaxation and sleep. Try to avoid chocolate, cheese, eggplant, ham, potatoes, sugar, spinach, sausage, tomatoes, and wine before bedtime. These foods contain tyramine, which increases the release of norepinephrine, a brain stimulant.

Chamomile Relief
Chamomile has long been the classic tea for relaxation and tension. A strong cup before bed can surely help anyone sleep soundly and wake up feeling refreshed and ready to go.

What do I do when my throat and mouth get dry during a performance?

Coconut Water
Coconut water is a fabulous hydrator, and it is full of potassium helping you to stay energized as well. Unlike water, coconut water will not strip away the thin layer of mucus needed on the chords to keep them hydrated. Too much water can do this. Coconut water will help keep this layer of mucus intact.

Ginger
Keep a small piece of Ginger about the size of a quarter in a plastic bag. When you begin to feel dry, slightly chew on the ginger. It will activate your salivary glands and coat your throat, keeping your vocal mechanism moist while you perform.

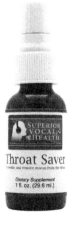

Throat Saver Spray
Throat Saver from Superior Vocal Health is designed to help remove excess mucus from the throat and open up the sinus passages with organic peppermint oil. It is also used to help keep the throat and cords moist. Throat Saver contains Xylitol, a natural berry extract that promotes salivation in the mouth and throat. This spray can be used all day long and can be purchased directly from the website, superiorvocalhealth.com.

It is my sincere desire and wish that this book has helped you become a more conscious, healthy, strong, and successful voice professional. Our path is not an easy one. We are our instrument. We need to always be aware of the health of our voice. Please use this book wisely and constantly to help you maintain, strengthen, and heal your body and voice naturally.

For continual postings and information on Natural Voice Care as well as the latest herbs, diet and supplements for your voice and body, subscribe to my blog at Superiorvocalhealth.com.

In addition you can "like" our Facebook page and stay up to date on new product releases and information from Superior Vocal Health.

Stay healthy, happy and whole.

As always, I wish you the best on your quest for Superior Vocal Health!

David Katz

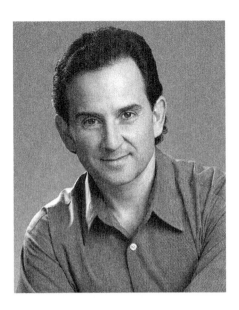

DAVID AARON KATZ is CEO and Founder of Superior Vocal Health. He is also a Cantor, nutritional consultant, herbalist and the author of the internationally read blog "Superior Vocal Health." He has been singing Opera and Broadway music internationally for more than 22 years.

He has sung with many prominent symphonies in the United States and Europe including the Pan American Symphony of New York, The Atlanta Symphony and the Houston Grand Opera Symphony with Marvin Hamlisch conducting. Mr. Katz has committed his entire career to helping fellow singers take care of their voices naturally without chemicals or drugs. Learn more at: Superiorvocalhealth.com.

CPSIA information can be obtained
at www.ICGtesting.com
Printed in the USA
BVOW06s1538050118
504329BV00001B/95/P